Michael J. McAndrew
III.

Spring 1974

Stay
of
Execution

Books by Stewart Alsop

STAY OF EXECUTION

THE CENTER

NIXON AND ROCKEFELLER

THE REPORTER'S TRADE (with Joseph Alsop)

WE ACCUSE (with Joseph Alsop)

SUB ROSA (with Thomas Braden)

Stay of Execution

A Sort of Memoir

by STEWART ALSOP

J. B. LIPPINCOTT COMPANY
Philadelphia and New York

The lines by T. S. Eliot quoted from "The Love Song of J. Alfred Prufrock," "Whispers of Immortality," and "Preludes," are from *Collected Poems 1909–1962* and are reprinted by permission of the publishers, Harcourt Brace Jovanovich, Inc.

The lines by Hilaire Belloc quoted from "Henry King" and "Jim" are from *Cautionary Verses* and are reprinted by permission of Alfred A. Knopf, Inc. *New Cautionary Tales* copyright 1931 by Hilaire Belloc; renewal copyright 1959 by Eleanor Jebb Belloc, Elizabeth Belloc, and Hilary Belloc. All rights reserved.

Photographs by Larry Keighley are reprinted with permission from *Saturday Evening Post* © 1956 The Curtis Publishing Company.

U.S. Library of Congress Cataloging in Publication Data

Alsop, Stewart, birth date
    Stay of execution.

        1. Leukemia—Personal narratives.   I. Title.
RC643.A39   362.1′9′61550924   [B]   73–13691
ISBN–0–397–00897–X

To Tish

Contents

A section of photographs follows page 160.

Preface

THIS is a peculiar book. I have two reasons, or excuses, for writing it. First, I have myself quite often wondered what it would be like to be told I had an inoperable and lethal cancer, and I suspect that a lot of other people have wondered the same thing. If a writer has had an unusual experience likely to interest a good many people, he has an instinct, and perhaps even a duty, to write about it.

Second, after I had been told my remaining span of life would be short, I began to think back quite often about the life behind me. This is in no sense an autobiography. But I hope it is more than a clinical record, and that the reader who gets bored—as any sensible person would—reading about hemoglobin or megakaryocytes or platelets will find some interest or amusement in reading about my odd war, or about my experiences as a journalist, or about some other experiences, and even some thoughts, I have had.

What partly makes this book peculiar is that my disease is peculiar. It was originally diagnosed as acute myeloblastic leukemia, or AML for short, which permits an average survival time of a year or a bit more. But it has, thank God, persistently refused to behave like acute myeloblastic leukemia.

9

There was one happy period, in the fall of 1971, when the doctors at the National Institutes of Health, where I have been treated, suspected that I didn't have cancer at all, but a sort of mimic cancer. Then, for some time, they suspected that whatever was wrong with me was a bizarre sort of cancer, totally atypical, perhaps a new disease—"Alsop's leukemia." As of this writing, the official diagnosis is "smoldering leukemia" or "aleukemic leukemia." This is a very rare kind of leukemia; there have only been about a dozen cases in NIH's history. Its chief difference from AML is this: Without chemotherapy, classic AML kills its victim in a few weeks. Smoldering leukemia may smolder on for years before breaking out into the lethal form of acute leukemia. My own guess is that this official diagnosis means that the doctors have decided I must have some form of leukemia, but they don't really know what kind it is or how long I am likely to survive it.

There is another reason this book is peculiar. It was all written by me, but it was written by different mes. Part of it was written by a me lying in bed in the leukemia ward at NIH in late July and early August 1971, waiting to be put into a "laminar flow room," to get chemical treatment which might buy me a year or so of life. Part of it was written by a me released from NIH in August with a question mark for a diagnosis, feeling pretty rotten, but not rotten enough to stop writing the column for *Newsweek* which is my chief source of livelihood and my chief reason for being as a journalist.

Part of it was written by a me feeling sick unto death in September, and indeed nearer to death than I realized at the time. Part of it was written a few weeks later by a euphoric me suddenly feeling better than I had for years and confident—or almost confident—of a final cure. And part of it

10

was written by a me—the me now writing—faced with a recrudescence of the mysterious disease and again in fear of an unwilling expedition to that "undiscover'd country from whose bourn no traveller returns."

This is, in short, a mixed-up sort of book. But I have led a mixed-up sort of life, and no experience of that life—not even when an American colonel almost had me shot as a German spy after I had parachuted behind the lines in France—has been more mixed up than the peculiar hell-to-heaven-to-purgatory existence I have had since I was first diagnosed as an acute leukemic. In a way, no experience has been more interesting than living in intermittent intimacy with the gentleman W. C. Fields used to call "the man in the white nightgown" and whom I have come to think of as Uncle Thanatos, and sometimes, when I have been feeling very sick, as dear old Uncle Thanatos. Death is, after all, the only universal experience except birth, and although a sensible person hopes to put it off as long as possible, it is, even in anticipation, an interesting experience.

11

Part One

AT ABOUT 9:30 on the morning of July 19, 1971, I suddenly knew that something was terribly wrong with me. I was standing on top of an old stone wellhead which we use as a dump at our country place in Maryland. The wellhead makes a fine dump. It has steep sides, topped by stone. The sides are about four feet high, and they conceal the trash from public view. There's plenty of room for the trash—it's still only about half full.

Dumping the trash is a predeparture ceremonial at our Maryland place, which is called Needwood Forest. July 19 was a Monday, and I was going back to work that day, after a fine three-week vacation. My four-year-old son, Andrew, brought out a couple of cardboard boxes to throw in the dump, and I carried a plastic pail filled with the weekend's rubbish. We clambered up the sides of the dump, which are steep and slippery, and Andrew threw in his boxes and I threw in the contents of the pail. Andrew shouted, "Come on, Daddy!" and scampered for the car. I couldn't move.

I had been feeling a bit tired lately, and I'd had trouble with shortness of breath. But I had never felt quite like this before. I was gasping like a fish on a beach, and I could hear my heart pounding furiously. It was all I could do, for a long moment, to keep my feet. "Face it, Alsop," I said to myself. "You're in trouble." (Later I remembered having said the same words to myself many years before.) Then I walked slowly to the car.

My wife, Tish, was at the wheel. She hardly ever lets me drive. She has a theory that I begin to think about politics, or something, and that then I let the car do the driving, which is dangerous. Eleven-year-old Nicky, our number five child, and Andrew, number six, were in the back seat. I said something about feeling sort of lousy, and Tish said something about its being lucky I had an appointment for a physical with Dr. Perry that afternoon, and we let the subject drop. As Tish drove us to Washington, the gasping and the pounding eased.

I married Tish in London during the Second World War, when she was eighteen and I had just had my thirtieth birthday. She was working for British Secret Intelligence at the time, though I didn't know about it until long after our marriage—British Intelligence was very strict about not telling foreigners *anything*. I was a lieutenant in a British regiment, the King's Royal Rifle Corps. One reason I had fallen in love with Tish, aside from the fact that she was beautiful, was that she was markedly undemonstrative. I found Tish's tendency to say nothing at all for long periods of time oddly entrancing. She is still laconic, especially where matters touching the emotions are concerned, and so am I.

This was one reason we said so little about the way I felt. Perhaps there was another reason too. When I was a small boy, I was sick a lot of the time—I had asthma and eczema and other unpleasant physical problems. But from my college days until that day I stood on the dump, I had never been seriously ill at all—I'd hardly ever had even a head cold. I was proud of never being sick, and like a rich man who thinks the poor must all be stupid, I tended to the notion that sick people were just weak-willed. When Tish had been sick, or when she had gone to the hospital to have a baby, I had been a bit cavalier about her troubles. Anyway, I couldn't believe that I was *really* sick.

By the time we arrived home I felt better, and I drove my own car downtown. At the *Newsweek* office I dictated some letters to my secretary, Amanda Zimmerman, who, being very pretty, very nice, and very competent, is the envy of journalistic Washington. Then I walked across Pennsylvania Avenue to lunch at the Metropolitan Club. I had a martini and a steak with two old friends, Philip Watts and Carl Gilbert—they both recalled later that I looked well and seemed merry as a grig. Then I walked the four blocks to Dr. Perry's office. Halfway there, I had the same sensation of dizzy breathlessness I had had on the dump that morning. I waited on a corner through two light changes before walking on.

Dr. Perry, the family doctor, is a competent and likable young man with a longish, faintly Lincolnian face. I had the usual tests and then sat in the waiting room, reading old copies of *Country Life*. A nurse summoned me to Dr. Perry's office. He looked graver and more Lincolnian than usual.

"You're anemic," he said. "You're *very* anemic. We've retested your blood six times, always with the same result. I want to get you into Georgetown University Hospital right away, this afternoon."

"Is it cancer?" I asked. I knew enough to ask that.

"That's not my first concern now," said Dr. Perry. But from his tone I could tell he had by no means ruled out cancer.

I walked to my car and drove the fifteen minutes to our Cleveland Park house. Tish was in the drive when I came in.

17

"Perry says that I'm very anemic and that he wants to get me into a hospital right away."

When I said this, Tish kissed me, suddenly and surprisingly. We hardly ever kiss in public, and, unlike couples much less happily married, we never call each other "darling," or even "dear." Tish knows a lot more about medicine than I do. She had worked in hospitals and for medical charities, whereas I had always felt about medicine and doctors as I had about hospitals—necessary, perhaps, but tedious and to be avoided at almost any cost. She knew enough to suspect strongly what I had only suspected vaguely—cancer.

Tish drove me to Georgetown University Hospital, and I registered as a patient at the front desk. As the various forms were being filled out, I spotted a slip with Dr. Perry's name on it and the notation: "Suspected aplastic anemia." I asked the lady at the reception desk what aplastic anemia was. She looked embarrassed, muttered something, and shuffled the slip under some other papers. Obviously I had not been intended to see it.

Upstairs, installed in a surprisingly comfortable room, I was visited by platoons of doctors, most of whom seemed to be in their twenties. They poked me, and pricked me, and drew blood out of me, and asked innumerable questions. The questions were often the same questions. Had I ever inhaled a lot of benzine? Did I swallow a lot of aspirin? Had I ever taken a drug called Chloromycetin?

The answer to all these questions was a tentative no. It was especially tentative in the case of the Chloromycetin. I remembered feeling very lousy indeed on a trip to Paris in 1969. I also remembered that the Hotel St. James et d'Albany's *valet de chambre*, a friendly fellow, had given me a big green cardboard tube filled with big white pills.

18

The green tube was covered with lettering boasting about the effectiveness of the pills against everything from *migraine* to *la grippe*. Three of the pills a day, the *valet de chambre* had promised, would fix me up in a jiffy. So, naturally, I had taken my three pills a day and soon began to feel better. Chloromycetin? Unlikely, but the French are pretty free and easy about drugs. Inquiries were later instituted by Paris friends, but we never found out what was in the green cardboard tube. I know now what an ass I was to take any unidentified and unprescribed pills at all.

At about nine that evening, I had my first bone-marrow test. A very young doctor came in, asked me to roll over on my stomach, and gave me a couple of shots of Novocain in the flat bony area at the bottom of the spine. Before I knew what he was doing, he poked a needle through the bone and into the marrow and sucked some marrow out. It was not unbearably painful, but it was very unpleasant—my legs jerked, like a frog's in a laboratory experiment.

The doctor turned the marrow over to a technician, who smeared it on slides and looked at it carefully.

"Enough spicules?" the doctor asked. That was a question I was to hear again. The technician said he thought he had enough, and the doctor told me that the marrow would be analyzed and that Dr. Perry would be in early the next morning to tell me the results.

"Will it show whether I have cancer?" I asked.

"Yes," said the young doctor confidently. "Whether you have cancer, and what kind." He didn't sound as though he had much doubt that I had cancer. He went out and left Tish and me alone. I was afraid and reached out for her hand, which felt warm and comforting and very much alive. Tish spent the night on a cot in the room beside my bed. Twice I woke up, despite the sleeping pill I had taken, and

19

was afraid and reached for Tish's hand. Both times she was awake.

The next morning, more young doctors came in to poke me and feel me and ask me questions. Then the visits stopped. Dr. Perry had been supposed to come in early with the verdict, but the hours dragged by and still no Dr. Perry.

Tish and I began telephoning the family to let them know where I was and what had happened. We started with my generation—my older brother Joe and his wife Susan Mary, my younger brother John and his wife Gussie, my sister, Corinne, who was also in a hospital. She had had a breast-cancer operation less than three weeks before.

Then we began calling the four eldest children. Number one, Joe, twenty-six, was an executive of a small computer company in Cambridge, Massachusetts. He wasn't in his office. Number two, Ian, twenty-four, was living in Katmandu, in Nepal. When he was fresh out of Dartmouth, where he had been an antiwar protester, he and I had gone to Vietnam together to have a look at the war. It was his idea to go—he was a cub reporter on a Virginia suburban paper at the time—and mine to go with him.

I thought it would be interesting to try to see the war through Ian's eyes, but in that sense the expedition was a failure. I don't think Ian ever quite decided what his eyes were seeing, though he wrote some good feature pieces for his paper. But we had a good time flying about in helicopters together. We said good-bye in the Hotel Caravelle in Saigon, and I left for home and he left to see a bit of the world. He had ended up in Katmandu, making a living selling Tibetan woodcut prints to tourists. It was a pretty good living, by Katmandu standards—he and his friend and partner, Jill, even had a working flush toilet in their house. We Alsops like to be comfortable.

Katmandu was not easily telephonable. So we called

our daughter, Elizabeth, who is married to Peter Mahony, an able architect, and was working as a children's book editor at Harper & Row. Elizabeth—"Fuff," she is called in the family, because when she was a very little girl Ian pronounced "Elizabeth" as "Fuff-fuff"—sounded sensible and reassuring, as she always does. Number four, Stewart, nineteen, was touring with two friends in a van, and we tried to reach him but failed.

Then we tried Joe again. Joe first demonstrated his competence as an electrical engineer by bugging the headmaster's study when he was a Fourth Former at Groton School —even the headmaster acknowledged that it was a technically impressive job. Joe was expelled, went to MIT, and then helped found a business in Massachusetts called Intercomp—International Computation, Inc. He expected to make a million right away. He hadn't made it yet, but a few months before, he had done something better when he married Candy Aydelotte, a charming blonde from Texas.

By the time we got Joe on the telephone, I had developed a sort of formula. I said I was in a hospital, and when Joe asked what was the matter, I said with an attempt at a laugh, "My blood seems to have turned to water."

There was no answering laugh, and quite a long pause. Then Joe said, "I love you, man."

Joe is perhaps the least demonstrative of our undemonstrative family. He is also anything but a fool, and he obviously knew that something must be very wrong. For the first time, I suddenly felt like crying, and I hung up quickly.

My brother Joe and Susan Mary came in, bearing fresh fruits and other viands, and words of good cheer. They then left, and Tish left briefly too, to get some magazines and papers, and I was alone for the first time. Suddenly I felt more lonely than I had ever felt in my life before.

About noon Tish came back—still no Dr. Perry. The

21

usual hospital lunch was wheeled in, perfectly edible but curiously unappetizing. Tish made me a martini—there is always plenty of cracked ice in a hospital—and it helped to give me some appetite and also to paper over the panicky suspense I had begun to feel.

Soon after lunch, Dr. Perry came in. There was something in his face—a sadly sympathetic air, a faint embarrassment—that smelled of bad news.

"I'm sorry," he said, and then I *knew* it was bad news, and I was glad I'd had the martini. "But you have leukemia. Acute myeloblastic leukemia."

"Are you sure I have this kind of leukemia?" I asked. I was rather proud that my voice was steady.

"Ninety-five percent sure," he said.

Then he explained that he had been promised a bed for me at the National Institutes of Health, "where they know more about leukemia than anywhere else in the world." Georgetown also had excellent leukemia specialists, he said, and of course, if I preferred, I could stay right there. I would be more comfortable at Georgetown, I would have a private room, and Tish could spend the night with me occasionally, whereas there were only double rooms at NIH. In either case I would be given a course of chemotherapy—a treatment with powerful chemicals to get rid of the malignant cells. At NIH I would probably be in a special room called a "laminar flow room," which reduced the risk of infection and thus increased the chance of successful treatment.

How long, I asked, would this treatment last? It could be as short as two weeks, said Dr. Perry, but it would be more likely to last a month or more. I hesitated a moment and then said I thought I'd better go to NIH.

I made the decision easily. In retrospect, I don't quite know why it was so easy. It wasn't money—I was fully insured, and I didn't know at the time that NIH was free. The room at Georgetown was a lot pleasanter than most hospital rooms, and the doctors seemed very able. I think it was partly that phrase of Dr. Perry's—"where they know more about leukemia than anywhere else in the world"—and partly the reputation of NIH, which, although I never paid any attention to such matters, I had unconsciously absorbed. A man who knows his life is in danger—and by this time I was of course aware that I was in danger of death—instinctively tries to better the odds.

The decision almost certainly prolonged my life. Chemotherapy, I discovered later, is a Rubicon. It buys the leukemia patient some time—if he is lucky, quite a lot of time—but it can also destroy whatever it is that enables the body to resist the leukemic cells. In the end death is certain. At Georgetown, I would have been put into a course of chemotherapy immediately. The chances are high that I would have had chemotherapy at NIH, too, if it hadn't been for Dr. John Glick.

The next day Tish drove me home from Georgetown to collect some clothes and books, and from there to NIH, a functional cluster of brick buildings mostly built in the mid-1950s during the Eisenhower administrations. We took the elevator to the thirteenth floor, on which the leukemia ward is inauspiciously located. Dr. John Glick was waiting for us there.

I got into bed in a small double room also occupied by an elderly farmer who had another kind of cancer. Tish sat in a chair by the bed, and Dr. Glick came in to talk to us. He sat down in another chair, beneath a reproduction of a Rouault painting of a woman—in the days to come I was to become drearily familiar with that Rouault.

Dr. Glick seemed surprisingly young, but I was already used to that—some of the doctors who had examined me at

Georgetown looked like college freshmen. He was very thin, with sideburns, a white coat, a tie and blue button-down shirt, and a quick, eager manner. It was very soon clear that he was highly intelligent, highly competent, and—this can be even more important to a patient whose life is at risk—a nice man and a good man.

The reason Dr. Perry had seen me so late, Dr. Glick said, was that the doctors at Georgetown had spent most of Tuesday morning arguing about my marrow slide. The Georgetown marrow slide was so unusual that he intended to give me another marrow test that evening, and there would be more after that.

The marrow was "hypocellular," he said—meaning that it had very few cells of any sort, normal or abnormal. According to the Georgetown count, about 44 percent of my cells were abnormal, and, he added, with a candor I later discovered was characteristic, "they're very ugly-looking cells." Most of them looked like acute myeloblastic leukemia cells, but not all—some of them looked like the cells of another kind of leukemia, acute lymphoblastic leukemia, and some of them looked like the cells of still another kind of marrow cancer, not a leukemia, called dysproteinemia. And even the myeloblastic, or AML, cells didn't look *exactly* like AML cells.

There was another puzzling thing about my case, Dr. Glick said. In the typical acute leukemic case—not all cases, of course—the malignant cells filled the marrow almost to bursting, enough to make the shinbones ache, and the white blood count was very high. Also, usually, there were abnormal cells in the blood. I had comparatively few cells of any sort, good or bad, and my white blood count was very low. There were no abnormal cells in the blood, only in the marrow.

Meanwhile, the diagnosis was acute myeloblastic leukemia, or AML. He had been assigned to my case, he said, and we would be seeing a lot of each other.

Then he gave me a head-to-toe physical examination, peering into my eyes with a sort of jeweler's magnifying glass, thumping me all over and asking me if it hurt, feeling under my ribs for my spleen and my liver, feeling in my armpits for swollen lymph glands, and so on. While this was going on, he asked me all the question I'd been asked at Georgetown and a lot of new ones, and I asked him some questions in the intervals.

How old was he? Twenty-eight. How long had he been at NIH? Only about three weeks. Was he married? Yes. Children? One on the way. All this between thumps and questions about benzine and Chloromycetin and how long I had been feeling badly. When I told him that I had had trouble with breathlessness and heart-pounding at least since early spring and maybe longer, he seemed interested and asked me a lot of questions, trying to pin down just when these symptoms had first appeared.

I told him that I remembered one time, in the late summer of the year before, when I'd played one set of tennis and had felt so awful from breathlessness and heart-pounding that I'd had to sit down. I'd been playing at Needwood with Tish against Rowland Evans and his wife, Kay. Evans is a friend and fellow columnist and a much better tennis player than I am. I've always wanted to beat him, and we almost won that set. Then I sat under a beech tree, feeling dizzy, with my heart pounding furiously, wondering if I was going to die. At the time, I ascribed my symptoms to the sun, advancing age, and my disappointed ambition to beat Evans. Then I remembered another time, at the opening of the dove season in September, when I set off with my old Winchester 12-gauge shotgun to a place about a half mile up the road from Needwood where I'd seen a lot of doves. I'd

25

suddenly felt so awful that I'd had to sit down and then turn back.

During the winter, I told Dr. Glick, and increasingly in the spring, I'd been really bothered with breathlessness, especially when I tried to rush the net at tennis. Dr. Glick seemed genuinely interested in all this. He seemed particularly interested in my left shinbone. I have played a lot of tennis since I was a boy, rather incompetently but with a lot of competitive spirit. I like to claim that I have "the arrogant grace of the great natural athlete," but when I serve, I often inadvertently hit my left shinbone with my racket, which great natural athletes don't often do. So my left shinbone looked like a rather bloody battlefield, with many old scars healed over. There was one new and unhealed scar on my knee, which is higher than I usually hit myself when I serve.

How long had this been going on? Dr. Glick asked. Oh, I'd been hitting myself with my racket for a long time, I said. It never really hurt, only lately it had seemed to bleed a lot—I supposed it was because I'd got a new steel racket, which opened the skin more than my old wooden racket. How much did it bleed when I hit myself? Well, lately it had become a sort of joke with the people I played with—my left leg would be covered with blood, and they would make unkind jokes about "the arrogant grace of the great natural athlete" and so on.

Dr. Glick explained why he was interested in my left shinbone. Cells called "platelets" control bleeding, he said, and a low platelet count, like a high white-blood-cell count, is characteristic of leukemia. My platelet count was very low, so the bloodied shinbone might provide evidence of how long I'd had leukemia.

That first day, John Glick was very impersonal and professional, but I liked him instinctively, and so did Tish.

26

Later, liking grew into affection and admiration and also into genuine friendship, a relationship not easily attained between a twenty-eight-year-old and a man twice his age.

Dr. Glick had asthma as a boy (as I did), and he has the slightly hunched shoulders of many asthmatics. He has a thin, sallow, interesting, and obviously intelligent face, and a certain unselfconscious intensity of manner. He has a good sense of humor, but when he is chasing after clues on which to base a diagnosis, he has the humorless intensity of a bloodhound on the trail. Even that first day, it seemed to me that he was genuinely interested in my case, perhaps in part for the same reason that Sherlock Holmes, after a long diet of easy solutions, would find a really difficult case so stimulating that he felt no need of his usual dose of laudanum.

John Glick is at once a very kindly and a very candid man, and for a doctor dealing with leukemics that is an uncomfortable combination. I asked him what was likely to happen to me, and he told me that I would probably be given chemotherapy to induce a "remission." The chemicals were very powerful, he said—"in fact, we call them poisons, and that is what they are." They killed the bad cells, but they killed a great many of the good cells too. I recalled that a doctor at Georgetown had said that the problem of treating leukemia was like trying to kill the crabgrass without killing the grass, and Dr. Glick said that was about right. During chemotherapy, the red blood cells and the platelets could be maintained at safe levels by transfusions, he said, but there was no sure way to maintain the white blood cells at a satisfactory level. They were the body's protection against infection, so infection during chemotherapy was the main danger to a leukemic's life.

That was why I'd probably end up in a laminar flow room, a kind of hospital room that existed at NIH but not at

27

Georgetown. In a laminar flow room, the air flowed only one way. It was pumped in from the outside, through the room, and into the hospital. At the thirteenth-floor level, there was virtually no danger of infection from the outside air, whereas the hospital air was likely to contain sources of infection. The patient, of course, never left the room until he was in remission and his white cells were back at a safe level. Doctors and nurses treated him with rubber gloves through a transparent plastic wall, and everything was sterilized—sheets, clothes, medicine bottles, everything.

"Can you sterilize martinis?" I asked. The laminar flow room sounded horrible.

"Yes," Dr. Glick said with a smile. "But you won't feel at all well while you're under treatment, even with martinis. After every five days of treatment we give you a rest for a few days, and then you'll feel better." Patients who went into the laminar flow room were chosen by lot, he said—I might get my treatment in an ordinary room, like this one, but the rate of infection was statistically lower in a laminar flow room. Either way, my hair, or most of it, would probably fall out, and I'd lose a lot of weight during chemotherapy. But the weight came back during a successful remission, and as for the hair—"We have a fine collection of wigs at NIH."

What were the chances of a successful remission?

Better than 50 percent, he said. This gave me pause. A lot of patients in the laminar flow rooms clearly left the rooms one way only, like the air. A person in remission could lead a "normal life," Dr. Glick said—I could go back to my job, and I might even be able to play tennis again.

How long would a remission last?

"We have an AML patient right here in the hospital tonight," he said cheerfully. "He's been in remission for seven years, he's just had his first relapse, and with chemo-therapy he's back in remission already."

But what was the average?

"About fifty percent of our patients with AML who go into remission last a year or more," he said, still trying to sound cheerful.

How many died before two years?

Dr. Glick hesitated a moment. "About ninety-five per-cent," he said, and briskly changed the subject.

That evening Dr. Glick gave me a marrow test, the first of many I have had at his hands. Instead of being taken by surprise in my bed, as at Georgetown, I was led into a treatment room in one of those hospital gowns open at the back, which seem to be designed to make the patient feel as unhappy and humiliated as possible. There were a couple of nurses and a male technician in the room. I lay down on my stomach, and Dr. Glick swabbed off my lower back and said, "This is the Novocain. It will feel like a mosquito bite." Then he stuck a needle into me.

"Mosquito bite, hell," I said. "It feels like a bloody great wasp."

"Okay," he said, "A wasp. Now here's another wasp, to get in a little deeper." This second needle, because of the Novocain, didn't hurt so much.

He waited a bit more and then went in again, with a third needle. I could feel it go through the bone and into the marrow, and I could feel the pull as he drew some marrow out. Again, as at Georgetown, it didn't really hurt all that much, but it was unpleasant, and my legs jerked again like a frog's.

There was a little delay as the technician did things with slides. "Sorry," the technician said, "no spicules."

"We'll have to go in again, with a bigger needle," said

29

Dr. Glick. "This won't take a minute." I could feel the needle go in again, and this time it hurt more.

"Got enough spicules?" Dr. Glick asked.

"Well, it may be enough," said the technician. "It's pretty thin,"

Dr. Glick said that we'd leave it at that for the time being, and that he would do another marrow the next morning. "We'll try to get a biopsy too," he said.

Spicules, he explained, were bits of marrow with fat in them, which gave a representative sample of the marrow cells. Without enough spicules, the slide might give a wrong picture of what was really going on in the marrow. It was particularly important to get spicules when the marrow was, as in my case, hypocellular, or very thin in all kinds of cells. I was glad for the respite. Being "marrowed"—the noun is used as a verb—is somehow psychically demeaning.

That night was a bad night. Tish went home about ten. Dr. Glick had prescribed a sleeping pill, and I sneaked another I had in my shaving kit and slept for about four hours. It must have been about two in the morning when I woke up. The little room was pitch dark, and my roommate, in the next bed, snored lightly. I thought first about the marrow test, next morning, and the way my legs would jerk like a frog's. Then I thought about what Dr. Glick had told me.

Would it really be worthwhile to spend a month or more cooped up all alone in a laminar flow room, losing my hair and my flesh, either to die in the room or to emerge a bald skeleton and wait for death? Would it not be more sensible to reach for Hamlet's "bare bodkin," in the shape of a bottle of sleeping pills? And then a sense of the reality of death crowded in on me—the end of a pleasant life, never to see Tish or Andrew or Nicky or the four older children again, never to go to Needwood again, or laugh with friends, or see the spring come. There came upon me a terrible sense of aloneness, of vulnerability, of nakedness, of helplessness. I got up, and fumbled in my shaving kit, and found another sleeping pill, and at last dozed off.

I never again had a night as bad as that night, nor, I think, shall I ever again. For a kind of protective mechanism took over, after the first shock of being told of the imminence of death, and I suspect that this is true of most people. Partly, this is a perfectly conscious act of will—a decision to allot to the grim future only its share of your thoughts and no more.

My brother John sent me *Uncle Fred in the Springtime* by P. G. Wodehouse, and my brother Joe sent me *The Duke's Children* by Anthony Trollope. Wodehouse and Trollope are old favorites, and I'd read both books before. But both Wodehouse and Trollope are marvelously re-readable, and Uncle Fred and the Duke of Omnium got me through the first few evenings, after Tish left—I'd read till the sleeping pill began to take effect and then doze off.

The conscious effort to close off one's mind, or part of it, to the inevitability of death plays a part, I suspect, in the oddly cheerful tone of much of what I've written in this book. I instinctively preferred, for example, to recall episodes that had amused me during the war, like my first meeting with Tish, rather than the times when I was unhappy or afraid. In the same way, I remembered from my career as a journalist those episodes that amused me, rather than those to which some profound meaning might be attached.

The protective mechanism is also an unconscious reaction, I think. I remember seeing much the same process at work in combat. There is the first sudden shock of realizing

31

that the people on the other side are really trying to kill you. On my first day at the front in Italy, I wandered down a path with Deering Danielson, another American in the British army. I remember looking up and seeing a couple of planes maneuvering above us—and then diving for a ditch as the bullets smack-smacked on the earth near us; and the sudden incredulous awareness that Deering and I—good old Deering and inoffensive Stew—were the targets of the bullets. But the incredulity soon wears off, and a kind of unhappy inner stolidity takes over, coupled with a strong protective instinct that the shell or the bullet or the mine will kill somebody else—not me.

In this way the unbearable becomes bearable, and one learns to live with death by not thinking about it too much.

MY MOTHER DIED on June 23, 1971. My sister, Corinne Chubb, had a breast-cancer operation on July 3. I got my acute leukemia diagnosis on July 20. Those were not good weeks for the Alsop family.

My sister is married to a very able and successful insurance executive, Percy Chubb, Chairman of the Executive Committee of the Chubb Corporation. Like me, she has six children, and she and Percy also have such pleasant appurtenances as a big place in New Jersey, a yacht, and half of a beautiful island in the Caribbean. She is the second oldest of the four of us, after Joe.

To her brothers, my sister has always been "Sis," and she seems to us to have changed less than we have. As a child, she was given to a disconcerting candor and fanciful ideas—a curious combination—and she still is. When we were children, Sis used an interesting device to dominate her brothers. She invented a rodential regent called Helen Ratty, who presided over "Helen Ratty's Kingdom," a saucer-shaped depression in the woods above our house in Avon, Connecticut. Whenever she wanted her way, Sis would say solemnly, "Helen Ratty wants . . ." Whatever Helen Ratty wanted was, of course, the word of law to the rest of us.

Sis had been home from the hospital for a few days, and I was still in NIH, when she telephoned me to tell me her theory of what was going on in heaven. She spoke with the same tone of authority she had used to give us the word from Helen Ratty's Kingdom. Mother, Sis said, had asked for a little chat with God. She had told God that she did not want her son Stew or her daughter Corinne to join her in heaven yet; she would tell Him when the time had come. God, of course, had agreed to put off the reunion.

Sis's theory struck me as sound. Mother was not a pretty woman—she had a bigger nose than any of us, which is a lot of nose—but she had an amazing self-assurance and a lot of charm. The self-assurance derived from the charm, I think, because the charm made it possible for her almost always to get her way. The charm in turn derived from the fact that she was a woman much involved in life, with a deep and entirely genuine interest in other people.

When we were young, an old friend of Mother's, Mrs. Ernest Lindley, told us the story of how, as a girl, Mother charmed Lord Dunsany, an Anglo-Irish aristocrat and man of letters, who was immensely tall, immensely distinguished, and immensely silent. My grandmother, who was the sister of President Theodore Roosevelt and a famous hostess of her era, gave Lord Dunsany a big dinner party in New York.

A very pretty and highly intelligent girl on the great man's right had been straining every nerve to get him to talk, but Lord Dunsany responded only with long, painful silences. When Mother's turn came, she shifted right around in her chair to face Lord Dunsany, put both elbows on the table, smiled worshipfully, and asked, "Where did genius begin?" Thereafter, according to Mrs. Lindley, it was impossible to get the great man to stop talking.

When Mother was expressing sympathy or interest a little too enthusiastically, we would turn around, put our elbows on the table, and ask, "Where did genius begin?" This made her laugh and damped her down a bit, but not for long.

During her last year, when she was eighty-four, she had constant pains in her stomach—the doctors never did find out just what was wrong—and the flame of her life flickered. Sometimes, briefly, there was the old gaiety and the deep involvement in other people's lives, but more and more rarely. Mother knew she was going to die and said more than once that she hoped it would be soon. It was a sad last year. Macbeth said of Lady Macbeth, "She should have died hereafter." Mother should have died herebefore. That is true, I suppose, of many old people. As de Gaulle said, old age is a shipwreck.

But until her last year or so, the remarkable self-assurance and the charm remained at full strength. Both were displayed in her relationship with her first cousin and childhood friend, Eleanor Roosevelt, and her much more distant cousin, President Franklin Roosevelt.

I recall vividly—all too vividly—a wartime incident which illustrated that relationship. I volunteered to join the British army shortly before Pearl Harbor. This was not as idealistic as it sounds. I had been turned down by the draft and all three services, because of asthma and high blood pressure, and then the draft board informed me it was considering reclassifying me as fit for "limited service." I saw myself folding towels in some damnable camp in South Carolina, while my friends were seeking the bubble reputation even in the cannon's mouth and having a lot of fun. I had heard from my younger brother John that a British regiment, the King's Royal Rifle Corps, which had originated in colonial America as the 60th Royal Americans, was taking a few American volunteers. So I went to the British Embassy in Washington and asked to see the military attaché.

I was ushered into the office of a tall, thin major with an enormous mustache. I told him that one reason I wanted to join the 60th Rifles, as the King's Royal Rifle Corps was called informally, was that I had been turned down on medical grounds by our own services.

"Eyes all right?" he asked. I said they were 20–20, and he told me not to worry about getting into the 60th Rifles— he'd arrange to get me onto a freighter in a convoy one day soon. He did have a bit of advice for me, though, he said.

"Be sure to take a dinner jacket, and a shotgun for the grouse season. And, if you can manage it, ship over a small runabout—very useful for weekends."

He was a bit out of touch, as I discovered some months later, when I arrived at the 60th training depot in Winchester, Hants. I slept on the floor, on a straw mattress called a "palliasse," ate cold porridge, and as a mere rifleman, or private, had no use at all for a dinner jacket, a shotgun, or a runabout.

One day, while I was doing drill—I was terrible at it —I was summoned from the parade ground to a pay telephone and was astonished to hear the voice of Ambassador John Winant. Mrs. Roosevelt, he said, had come on a visit to England, and my mother had asked her to be sure to look me up and report on my state of mind and health. So could I come to tea the next day at the Embassy?

The 60th Rifles had a way of instilling in a rifleman a proper degree of humility, and I felt very humble at tea, surrounded by Ambassador Winant, Ambassador Tony Biddle (who was in uniform, with so many ribbons that they went over his left shoulder), various intimidating people with titles, and the President's wife. I was sitting in an armchair in embarrassed silence when Cousin Eleanor (as I had called her since I was a little boy) handed me a cup of tea. As I reached over to take it, the brass buttons on the fly of my battle dress burst from their moorings and rolled across the floor. There was a moment of silence, as all eyes followed one brass button, which continued to roll interminably. Then, in a kindly effort to cover my confusion, the President's wife asked me whether the British troops appreciated Spam, a kind of horrid fake ham which was a major item of Lend-Lease. I blurted out the tactless truth—that they hated the stuff—and then retired in confusion, my hand held over my private parts.

Mother thought nothing of asking her first cousin to do so small an errand for her—what were families for? Since she had seconded the nomination of Alf Landon in 1936 and made many anti-New Deal speeches, it took a certain brass for her to ask favors of the President, but it never bothered her at all. Twice during the war she called Pa Watson, the President's secretary, and politely demanded a "little chat" with the President. Once was when she wanted to make sure that my brother Joe would be on the Japanese prisoner exchange list—the Japanese had captured him when they took Hong Kong, and he was in the Stanley prison camp there. The other time was when the American army had refused to accept my transfer from the British army.

Both times Mother had her way in the end. And both times the "little chat" went on for more than an hour. The President liked Mother, despite her politics, and he was sentimental about old times. I don't suppose he ever knew that, when he was courting Eleanor in Dark Harbor,

Eleanor's young cousin Corinne always referred to him as "the Featherduster" in her diary and repeatedly expressed the hope that "darling Eleanor" would not marry him, with his "narrow shoulders" and "his eyes too close together."

It was natural to imagine Mother, when Sis and I got into trouble, calling on Saint Peter and asking for a "little chat" with God. After Sis told me her theory, I got into the habit, when seized with the fear of death, of making a small prayer: "Please Mother, please God." Eventually, I added two more people in heaven I had loved, my father and my Scottish nurse Aggie Guthrie, who nursed me through a sick childhood, so that the prayer became standardized: "Please God, please Mother, please Father, please Aggie."

W

"HAT ARE THE COUNTS?" Or: "Your platelets are holding up okay, but your granulocytes are in the cellar, I'm sorry to say." Or: "Your hemoglobin is around nine point five. But don't worry—if it goes below nine we'll transfuse you and bring you back over eleven." Or: "There's an increase in the megakaryocytes in your marrow, but I've got to say I couldn't find many granulocytic precursors." Or: "Now, don't get excited. But the percentage of blasts in your marrow is down from around forty percent to around twenty-eight percent. Probably just a blip on the screen—but it sure isn't bad news."

Before I got sick, all this would have been gobbledygook to me, but after the first week or so at NIH I spoke this new language like a native. After I understood the meaning of the blood counts and the less frequent marrow tests, I would wait for the results—as all leukemics do—with a fast-beating heart. For they can spell life, or death.

In retrospect I am astonished how little I once knew about the blood and about the function of the marrow. A tiny drop of blood at the end of your finger can show quickly, under a microscope, how energetic you are, how you would bleed if badly cut, what defenses you have against infection, and all sorts of other things.

39

Every morning, patients in Ward 13 of NIH would get a "finger stick" to provide that revealing drop of blood. A cheerful lady with faded blond hair—she told me she had been pricking fingers for a living for fifteen years—would come around every morning at about eight, ask you which finger you wanted pricked that morning, and then jab a little needle into that finger, skillfully and almost painlessly. Then she would squeeze the blood into thin plastic tubes and onto glass slides, and move on with a cheerful word to another leukemic.

About four hours later, after the technicians had analyzed the blood, peering at the slides through powerful microscopes or using expensive machines operating on a centrifugal principle, the patient would be told "the counts." A patient with good counts would feel bucked up for the day. Bad counts were bad news—much worse news than the gloomiest headlines in the newspapers.

My counts when I entered NIH were: hemoglobin, 6.8; platelets, 18,000; white blood count, 1,100 with 14 percent granulocytes. I once asked John Glick what these figures really meant, and he went into details about cells per cubic centimeter and the like. What he said would no doubt have interested my mathematical son Joe, but I have never been able to balance my checkbook, and he soon lost me. The mathematics don't interest the leukemic anyway. What matters to him is how far he is away from death. Although I'd played tennis the weekend before and had waded across the upper Potomac to fly-fish for small-mouth bass four days earlier, those first counts meant that I was quite close to being dead.

Hemoglobin supplies energy, *élan vital, joie de vivre.* If you have a high hemoglobin count—lots of red blood cells —you're in a mountain climbing or girl-chasing mood. "An inability to think, a strong desire to doze and drink"—G. K. Chesterton's heroic couplet (or is it Hilaire Belloc's?) sums up the way a person with a low hemoglobin count feels.

A man can carry on somehow—"to grunt and sweat under a weary life"—with a hemoglobin count of 10 or so. I suspect, and so does John Glick, though there's no way to prove it, that my hemoglobin count had been far under normal for as much as a year before I went to NIH. For years I have liked to have a brief snooze in the afternoon (so did Napoleon Bonaparte, Winston Churchill, Lyndon Johnson, and for that matter John F. Kennedy, who was younger than I). Part of my agreement with *Newsweek,* when I switched from the *Saturday Evening Post* in 1968, was that I would have a sleepable-on couch in my office. That last year before I went to NIH my snoozes became longer and longer; every afternoon I would get almost unbearably sleepy, close my door, lie down, and go into a catatonic state.

A normal hemoglobin count is between 14 and 16, and the closer to 16 the more *joie de vivre.* When a person's red blood count goes below 8, he is in danger of congestive heart failure. To supply sufficient energy—giving hemoglobin to the lungs and the rest of the body—the heart has to work overtime, and under sufficient stress it just gives up, like a furnace that explodes or simply goes out when it can't meet the demands placed on it.

My breathlessness and the heavy beating of my heart before I went to Dr. Perry's office were outward and visible signs of a low hemoglobin count. With a count of 6.8, I was lucky I didn't die on the tennis court or in the middle of the upper Potomac. But a low red blood count can be temporarily corrected in a few hours with a hemoglobin transfusion. John Glick stuck a needle in a vein the first night I

41

was in NIH, hung a bag of blood on a metal contraption called an "I.V."—for intravenous—and fed it into my blood stream. The bags vary, but they average about two pints. After four bags I felt full of beans—fuller of beans than I had for a good many weeks.

A doctor does not like to transfuse his patients any more than necessary, though. With every four bags of blood (except frozen blood) there is about a 1.5-percent chance of hepatitis. A patient who has had a lot of transfusions is lucky if he has not caught hepatitis, and a patient with both leukemia and hepatitis, for which there is no specific cure, is not at all a good insurance risk. Ways of screening out hepatitis have been improved constantly, but the screen is not yet 100 percent safe. Blood from commercial blood banks is the riskiest. People who make an extra buck selling their blood are almost by definition poor people, and the poor are more likely to have dormant hepatitis than people who volunteer their blood.

Red blood transfusions were first performed around the turn of the century; they were the first true body transplants. Since then techniques for matching blood precisely to avoid rejection have been perfected. Platelet transfusion is a much more recent technique, for which Dr. Isaac Djerassi (of whom more later) deserves a big share of the credit. Platelets are the cells that cause clotting and prevent a man from bleeding to death if he is cut. Death from hemorrhage was the most likely exit for a leukemic before platelet transfusion techniques were invented. Now it is rare.

Platelet counts vary widely. A low normal would be around 160,000, but some people have platelet counts of 400,000 or more. A level of 20,000 is considered the danger point. John Glick also gave me two bags of platelets right away, and my count briefly jumped from 18,000 to 34,000,

42

then rapidly sank back to around 18,000 again. Platelet transfusions are four times as likely to cause hepatitis as red blood transfusions, because it takes four bags of red blood to make one bag of platelets.

The platelets were why John Glick was so interested in the old scars on my left leg, where I had been hitting myself with my tennis racket so constantly. The scars not only suggested that I had had a low platelet count for a long time. They also suggested that even with a low count I did not hemorrhage easily. An episode that had happened the weekend before I was hospitalized, which I described to Dr. Glick, pointed to the same conclusion.

I had taken a fly rod down to the pond—it is really hardly more than a puddle—at Needwood, to fly-fish for bluegills. After catching some small bluegills, I climbed over a rusty fence to go back to the house and scratched my bottom and left leg badly. It was a long, deep cut, and I bled a lot, but I had the minimum common sense to wash the cut thoroughly, and in time the bleeding stopped. This too suggested to John Glick that I could manage on a low platelet count—otherwise the long scratch might have killed me.

My hemoglobin and my platelets were both in the danger zone, but my white blood count—1,100 with 14 percent granulocytes—was even more dangerously low. The white blood cells are the cells that fight off infection. It is their fierceness on the attack against alien cells that makes body transplants so difficult.

There are several different kinds of white blood cells, but for a leukemic the most important are granulocytes. The granulocytes are the principal battlers against infection. So when a doctor asks for "the WBC"—white blood count— he expects to be told not only the total count but the percentage of granulocytes. A normal WBC would be 4,000

43

to 10,000 white cells, with 45 percent to 75 percent granulocytes. A count of 500 granulocytes is the minimum safety level, though the prognosis is a lot better if a patient's granulocyte count is over 1,000. With a count of 500 granulocytes, the body can at least put up some sort of fight against infection. With less than 500, the body has very little fight left. When I entered the hospital, my granulocyte count was about 150. My lack of fight soon became apparent.

I entered NIH from Georgetown Hospital on Wednesday, July 21, and on Friday, after blood and platelet transfusions and two marrow tests, John Glick made a difficult decision. This was the decision not to put me into chemotherapy but instead, for the time being at least, to do nothing—to send me home and keep an eye on me.

Dr. Glick and Dr. Edward Henderson, the chief of the leukemic section, and the other doctors agreed by a big majority that I had AML, although there was one holdout for acute lymphoblastic leukemia and another for dysproteinemia. But to John's intuitive medical eye there was something so fishy-looking about the abnormal cells in my marrow, and something so unusual about my case, that he decided to wait and see, rather than put me right into chemotherapy and the laminar flow room. There were risks involved in the decision, of course. The greatest risk was that I might die of infection because of my defenseless state. But such risks had to be balanced against a near certainty—that if I had chemotherapy I would die, probably within a year, almost certainly within two.

John Glick had told us that I could go home on Saturday. On the afternoon of Friday, July 23, I convened a small business meeting. My younger brother, John, who is President of the Covenant Group of Insurance Companies and is the businessman of the family, had flown down from Hart-

44

ford. My old friend and broker Philip Watts joined us, and the three of us conferred solemnly about the changed family financial prospects, given the statistical probability that I would be dead in a year or a bit more.

We were calm and businesslike as we counted up my assets and discussed the need for a new will, for selling my two houses (but not on a forced-sale basis), for reinvestment for maximum income rather than growth to provide adequately for Tish, and so on. It gave me an odd sense of unreality—it was hard to grasp that it was, after all, *my* death we were discussing so rationally, and I had a feeling that we were three characters in a rather bad play. Then, as the discussion wound to an end and we poured Scotch and sodas, I began to have another feeling. It was midsummer and the anteroom we had co-opted for our discussion was air-conditioned. But it seemed to me that somebody must have turned the air conditioning way up. I kept shivering and asked a nurse for a blanket. By the time we had finished our Scotches, I was shivering uncontrollably. I had a chill— my first chill, as far as I can remember, but not my last.

That night my temperature went to 102, and on Saturday morning it was up to 104. By Saturday afternoon, instead of going home, I was attached via a vein in my right arm to two antibiotics, Keflin and gentamicin. They are very powerful—John Glick called them "cidal." Because my white cell count was so low, he explained, my defense against infection was inadequate, and I had some sort of infection which was causing my fever. The antibiotics would kill the infection, probably in a day or so, but to be sure the infection didn't recur it was necessary to keep me hooked up to antibiotics for ten days.

If my infection was due to a low white count, I asked Dr. Glick, why not give me a white cell transfusion, like the

45

hemoglobin and platelet transfusions he'd already given me? That was just the trouble, he said. White cell transfusions weren't like hemoglobin and platelet transfusions. They were possible—there had been a good many white cell transfusions at NIH—but it was very difficult to match the cells, and these transfusions often failed, because the existing white cells fought off the reinforcing cells as though they were invaders.

The only reliable white cell transfusions were from one identical twin to another. The next best was a transfusion from a sibling—not a child or a parent, but a brother or sister with the same genetic inheritance. If a sibling's white cells matched the patient's, a white cell transfusion usually succeeded. But the effects didn't last more than a day or so—white cells have a short half-life. And it was a risky business anyway.

Except *in extremis*, Dr. Glick explained, the cidal antibiotics were better weapons against infection than white cell transfusions, which were only used at NIH when they were just about the last hope. But of course the state of the art was improving all the time, and maybe the time would come when white cell transfusions would be as routine—and as life-sustaining—as platelet and hemoglobin transfusions.

Those first ten days at NIH, I also began to understand something about the purpose and meaning of the marrow tests. The basic purpose was to find what the malignant cells were up to—whether they were crowding out and killing the good cells and whether they were increasing or decreasing. Under a microscope, technicians carefully counted the percentage of abnormal cells in every marrow slide. But the marrow slides showed other things too.

Cells in the marrow produce cells in the blood. A big

reddish cell called a "megakaryocyte" is the "precursor" of the platelets, and there are hemoglobin and white cell precursors too. So an experienced doctor or technician, peering at a patient's marrow slides through a microscope, can make a pretty reliable estimate of what is happening—and what is going to happen—to the patient's blood. "Your hemoglobin should hold up all right," John Glick would tell me after peering at my marrow slides, "but your granulocytic precursors are very thin, and your megakaryocytes are substantially absent." Then I would know that my finger sticks would show sadly low platelets and granulocytes. John Glick was almost always right—but not always, for sometimes the besieged marrow can start churning out good cells for no precisely definable reason.

My sudden fever abated soon after I went on antibiotics. Until then, I had not felt especially sick, although I had been diagnosed as having terminal cancer. That Saturday morning when my temperature went up to 104, I was a sick man and knew it. After the antibiotics took effect and my temperature went down to normal, I again felt pretty well. Perhaps as a distraction from fear, I wanted to see people. We would have daily picnics, complete with martinis and occasionally wine, in one of the two large waiting rooms of Ward 13, to the surprise and occasional irritation of the nurses and the other patients. But although my temperature had disappeared within twenty-four hours, John Glick kept that damn needle in a vein for ten full days —it would fall out or get stopped up after a day or so and then have to be reinserted. He wanted to be 100 percent sure that whatever infection was attacking my nearly defenseless body was indeed dead.

Against the day when he might want a platelet transfusion or even a white-blood-cell transfusion from them,

47

John Glick asked for blood tests from my two brothers (Sis was eager to be tested, but Dr. Glick ruled her out because of her breast-cancer operation). My brother John turned out to have an entirely different sort of blood.

When we were little children, we used to be a bit nasty to John, as older children are to younger ones. We played two games, "Chase John" and "Run away from John." I can still remember John's chubby little legs running in both directions. We also invented the theory that John wasn't really an Alsop at all but a Bellotti. The Bellottis were a very nice Italian family who lived on our Connecticut tobacco and dairy farm, and it was true that John had a sort of family resemblance to Tony Bellotti, the chief of the clan, a stout man with a round, rubicund, cheerful face. John has the same kind of face. I wrote John, after the blood test, that this was the final proof that he was a Bellotti and not an Alsop at all.

Joe's test turned out to be a perfect fit. John Glick remarked that Joe's blood was fine, but a "bit old." Naturally, I could hardly wait to repeat this remark to my older brother. Fortunately, so far, I haven't had to call on him for his elderly white blood cells, but his elderly platelets have proved very useful indeed.

JOURNALISTS USUALLY acquire bad habits—indolence and a tendency to drink too many martinis, for example. I am a slave to both habits, but I have managed to acquire one good habit as well. Because I know how unreliable my memory is, I keep a notebook in my pocket or within easy reach at all times, and I spend a lot of time scribbling in it.

I feel naked without a notebook, and when one is filled I get another and start scribbling in it again. Being a pack rat by nature, I keep all my old notebooks—somewhere in Amanda Zimmerman's files (I have no idea how to find anything in them) notebooks are heaped like corpses on a battlefield, dozens and dozens of them. T. S. Eliot's Prufrock measured out his life with coffee spoons. I measure mine out with notebooks.

The notebook I had with me when I was hospitalized is about half filled with the raw material a Washington columnist uses to make his livelihood. Toward the beginning, there are notes about one of those "revolts" that are always going on in the State Department and never get anywhere: "Young Turks . . . Junior F.S.O. club. Union? AFL? Old Turks edgy. . . " Then the cryptic notation: "The

49

weakness is *us* . . . we don't have the Masada complex."
Masada is the mountain where the Jews of the second century died to the last man rather than surrender to the Roman legions. Somebody I had interviewed at the State Department had called the Israelis' stubborn, single-minded concern with their own security and survival their "Masada complex." This is not a complex that currently afflicts many Americans.

There are other scribbles, and then, at the top of a page, about halfway through the notebook, there is the word "leukemia."

This word was scribbled in my notebook on the morning of July 21, the day after Dr. Perry had pronounced my sentence. Then some more scribbles: "Amazing how nice almost everybody is. . . . God tempers the wind to the shorn lamb . . . old cliché . . . suddenly a vivid visual picture . . . *Horribilis mors perturbat me.* . . . *Perturbat* the right word . . . remission of sins . . ."

There are more scribbles, and then a few words that frightened me as much as I have ever been frightened by words. I can't remember just what day it was that I saw the words, but it was several days after my chill and fever, and I was still attached to the I.V. It was warm and sunny, and when Tish came in at about eleven one morning she suggested that we escape from the thirteenth floor for a while and go up to the solarium on the floor above, to smell a bit of fresh air and see the sun.

We took the elevator to the fourteenth floor, and as I pushed my I.V. in front of me, with the bottles of antibiotics dangling from it, we walked out into the open air. But the air was not all that open. The solarium was completely covered with a thick wire mesh, overhead as well as along the sides. The purpose, obviously, was to prevent suicides. There was something depressing about the wire mesh; it gave me a trapped feeling. Tish and I lay in the sun for a while, on folding cots, and I tried to read, but the sun was too bright. Restlessly, I got up to do some exploring. I wandered about, and came to a door off the solarium, and pushed it open, and found myself in an auditorium.

Then I saw the words that frightened me. There was a large placard on a stand, presumably for the indoctrination of newly arrived doctors and nurses. It was headed Rules for Admission, and there were ten or twelve numbered rules. I read only the first two: ALL PATIENTS MUST HAVE INCURABLE CANCER. ALL PATIENTS MUST BE INFORMED FRANKLY OF THEIR CASE.

I turned around quickly and shut the door. I said nothing to Tish, except that I wanted to go back to the room. Somehow those printed words brought home the reality to me in a way that all John Glick's kindly candor had not, and inside me there was a dark pit of fear. I can't talk about fear when I feel it, even with my wife. I can only talk about it when it's over.

One thing I discovered in those first ten days at NIH. A man can't be afraid all the time. No doubt if you were told that you were to die in three hours, you would spend those three hours being afraid of death. But when death is due to occur at some time in the fairly near but indefinite future—in a few months, or a year, or two years, or maybe even later—it is possible to forget about death for many hours at a time.

I suppose I first read the Latin tag scribbled in my notebook—*"Horribilis mors perturbat me"*—in about Third Form year at Groton, where I went to school in the Endicott Peabody era, when much Latin was compulsory. I remember thinking that "perturbed" seemed a rather mild reaction

51

to "horrible death." But it turned out to be, as I also scribbled, "the right word." Not that I wasn't afraid. I was, and I hated the idea of dying soon. But after the initial shock of being told that I had a lethal and inoperable cancer, the protective mechanism took over, so that for the most part I was perturbed—upset, worried—rather than terrified.

"God tempers the wind to the shorn lamb." I thought the words were from the Bible, until I looked up the phrase in Bartlett's and found it was Laurence Sterne's. And I did indeed have a "sudden visual picture"—of myself as the shorn lamb, naked to the cold wind; and the wind dying down as the protective mechanism took over, rendering the intolerable tolerable.

"Amazing how nice almost everybody is." A lot of the nurses wore on their shirt fronts those yellow plastic buttons with the outline of a fatuous grin, and almost all of them tried hard to cheer up their sure-to-die patients. Ward 13E, I discovered later, was not a popular ward with the nurses, and it was hard to keep it fully staffed. Taking care of leukemics is a lot of work. They have needles in their arms a good deal of the time, for chemotherapy or antibiotics or transfusions, and the needles are always getting clogged up or coming unstuck. They require a lot of care in other ways, especially the patients in the laminar flow rooms. But there was another reason 13E was unpopular. As one young nurse remarked to me, "Gee, this ward is just so *depressing*." So it is, but almost all the nurses did their very best to seem briskly cheerful.

The patients, for the most part, felt too horrible to be very genial. Some had just completed chemotherapy and were in the early stages of "remission." They looked deathly ill, with yellow-bronze parchment faces and wispy hair. But they too made an effort at cheerfulness, or at least at concealing despair. The word "cancer" was hardly ever mentioned, and the word "death" never.

"Remission of sins"—the phrase tantalized my memory for several days. The phrase was suggested, of course, by the "remission," alas temporary, which with luck followed a session of chemotherapy. I couldn't remember the rest of it, or where it came from. Finally, Tish supplied the rest: "remission of sins, resurrection of the dead, and life everlasting." From the Credo, of course.

Leafing through that notebook brought back to me vividly bits and pieces of those ten days at NIH. Tish would come in every day, usually at about eleven, go out in the afternoon to do errands, and then come back for dinner, with some agreeable tidbits to vary the monotony of the hospital diet. At first, her devotion made me feel a trifle guilty, since when she was in the hospital, usually with a new baby, I could rarely force myself to spend more than an hour with her, hating hospitals as I do. But I soon got used to her being there most of the day and resented it when she left me alone.

In fact, I more than resented being left alone—I feared it. On the second page of my notebook, after the scribble "leukemia," there is a longer scribble: "Tish left briefly this afternoon and suddenly I was alone with an awful loneliness." Those words tell something about what it is like to have a killing cancer, especially at first.

You become terribly dependent on other people, and the physical presence of other people becomes essential to you. Ordinarily, I rather like being alone, but on the rare occasions when I was alone during those first ten days at NIH I hated it. I was even thankful for my roommate, the elderly farmer who shared my room. We had very little in common, and he was presumably dying too, but at least he was a warm body.

Tish, thank God, could spend a lot of time with me, thanks to Nora and Olga, the invaluable El Salvadorians who live with us, and who kept an eye on Nicky and Andrew when Tish was at NIH. Tish asked me if I wanted Nicky and Andrew to visit me in the hospital, and I said I didn't. There is something demeaning about being in pajamas in daylight, in a hospital bed, hooked up to an I.V., surrounded by nurses and sick people, and I didn't want my children to see me demeaned.

At first my dependence on other people annoyed me. It more than annoyed me, it infuriated me. I hate being dependent and have fought against it all my life. Perhaps it is something in the genes.

I found out a bit about my genes in 1968. In that year, as its inevitable demise approached, the dear old *Saturday Evening Post* started a series on American families, in a futile attempt to recapture some of the old *Post* readership that had been lost by the editors' foredoomed attempt to appear "with it." The editors asked me to do a piece about my family, and I agreed. I'd never paid any attention to my ancestors before, although I was aware that I had a lot of them. I couldn't avoid being aware of them, since virtually without exception, on both sides, they had had their portraits painted, so that all the family houses, including my generation's, were festooned with ancestral portraits, some quite decorative, some hideous. But I'd never had any interest in these people in the gilt frames, or what they had done, until the *Post* asked me to do the family piece.

It wasn't a very good piece. The cast of characters ranged from a couple of Presidents to the family thief and a collateral murderer, and it was too complex. But I got an unexpected pleasure out of learning about my ancestors.

It gave me a comforting sense of being part of an unending continuum, of something that had started a long, long time before I was born and would go on for a long, long time after I was dead. And I found out some interesting things.

For one thing, not one of my direct ancestors, on either my mother's side or my father's, had ever taken any part whatever in any war. During the Civil War, Theodore Roosevelt's father, who was my great-grandfather, had been appointed to something called the Sanitary Commission, which was an elegant draft dodge. Perhaps that was why T. R. was so much the warrior. On the Alsop side, Joseph Wright Alsop III (my brother Joe is number five of that name, and my son Joe is number six) had "sent a man in his place," during the Civil War, and Joseph Alsop I had done exactly the same thing during the Revolution.

For another thing, not one of my ancestors had ever worked for any appreciable length of time in a position of salaried dependence. I think these two characteristics were related. It was not so much that my ancestors were cowards, though no doubt some of them were. They just hated the idea of being in a subordinate and dependent position—and nothing is more dependent and subordinate than an army recruit.

I suspect that I joined the 60th Rifles because of my genes. I had an irrational feeling that in a foreign army I would be more my own master, and if it turned out to be too intolerable I could just resign and go back home. My genes, I think (plus some small tax advantage), also explain why all my contracts with the *Post* and later with *Newsweek* identified me as an "independent contractor" rather than a salaried employee. This contractual provision has given me the wholly illusory feeling of being my own master, free to come and go as I please.

In any case, no doubt because of my genes, the condition of dependence to which being seriously ill reduced me was repugnant to me. I was dependent on the nurses. If I wanted a sleeping pill, or to have my bedclothes changed (I had night sweats every night while I was in the hospital), I had to ask a nurse. If a nurse woke me up to get weighed, I had to get up and get weighed. It was a bit like being a private all over again.

I was dependent—deeply dependent, and for my very life—on John Glick, and it was John, not I, who decided when I could have my I.V. removed (after ten days or so, an I.V. becomes a hateful encumbrance) or what treatment I should have, or whether I could go home and what I could do when I got there.

I was dependent above all on Tish, and in a way that I had not been dependent on any human being since Aggie Guthrie took care of me when I was very sick as a little boy. I was dependent on Tish not only for edible tidbits, martinis, books, and the like, but for a sort of unspoken emotional sustenance—for the squeeze of a warm hand in a time of darkness and fear. In time, I got used to this sense of dependence, and I even came, in a way, for the first time in my life, to enjoy it. Tish, knowing me, knew that I resented being dependent, and the emotional sustenance she gave me was therefore always unspoken.

I first met Tish in the summer of 1942, when I was an officer cadet in the King's Royal Rifle Corps. The OCTU— Officer Cadet Training Unit—was stationed in York, the lovely old cathedral town in northern England. There were five other Americans in the OCTU. One of them was a very handsome recent Harvard graduate, George Thomson, who was later best man at my wedding.

George, a man of great charm, was the social manager of the Americans in the KRRC. He had a genius for getting to know people, and within months he seemed to know half England, especially the much less than half England who owned the stately homes. Somehow, he had got an introduction to the Premier Baron of England, who owned a stately home not far from York. The Premier Baron is the baron whose ancestors were barons before any other baron's ancestors.

The Premier Baron was the Baron Mowbray and Stourton, and his stately home was called Allerton Castle. The Premier Baroness had written George, asking him to come for the weekend and to bring a friend. George had asked Harry Fowler, another American in the King's Royal Rifle Corps, whom we called Plowboy Fowler, because in those days he looked like a plowboy. (Now he looks like a bank president, which he is.) But Plowboy had been ordered on guard duty, so I went along as a substitute. If Plowboy hadn't been ordered on guard duty, my six children would not exist. Dreadful is the mysterious power of fate.

A KRRC officer who was some relation of the Premier Baroness had managed to wangle some petrol, and he drove us to the castle, which turned out to be an architectural disaster. A nineteenth-century Premier Baron had become disenchanted with the original Tudor castle, and he had torn the whole place down in the Victorian era and replaced it with a monstrous fake castle which looked very much like the fake castles the American robber barons used to build in New York City, on the Hudson, or in Long Island.

We approached the monstrous pile cautiously; there seemed no sign of life anywhere and no one answered our knockings. The Victorian glass on the front door was thick with dust, and George Thomson was wiping the dust off with his handkerchief to get a glimpse inside when the door was flung open and there stood the Premier Baron himself. He had bulging blue eyes, a baronial nose, and very little chin—in short, a baron straight out of Wodehouse.

"Who are *you*?" he asked, not very hospitably.

George started to explain, and the Baron, noting his accent, interrupted.

"Are you Americans?" he asked accusingly.

George said we were.

"Good God," said the Baron, profoundly moved. "Always had a rule here, back to my grandfather's time. No motor cars. No Americans."

He paused for a moment, obviously considering whether still another ancient tradition should be sacrificed.

"However," he said briskly, "here you are. Might as well come in."

Inside, we found a party in progress. The castle was to be taken over by the Royal Canadian Air Force within a few days, and this was a last fling. Of the once vast servant corps, only an ancient, arthritic butler remained, but the huge table in the banqueting hall groaned with grouse, fruit, vegetables from the garden, and the best claret and port from the cellar.

In a comfortable sitting room we had highly potable, very cold martinis—a surprise, for in those days the English version of a martini consisted of warm sweet Vermouth with a dash of gin. There was another, equally pleasant surprise—two pretty girls, both wearing a lot of lipstick and swilling down the martinis with enthusiasm. What with the lipstick and the gin, George and I thought they must be nineteen or twenty, a respectable age for us, since George was twenty-four and I was twenty-eight. One of the pretty girls was a Saxon blonde and clearly the daughter of the Premier Baron. The other—introduced as Tish, real name Patricia—had mouse-colored hair and attracted me strangely. As I later wrote the family, she looked like a Trollope heroine, one of the really nice ones.

I sat next to her at dinner. My hair had been cut very short—the British army's idea, not mine—and her first remark to me was, "You look like a criminal." This seemed an intriguing start, but after that I could hardly get her to say more than "Please pass the salt," which intrigued me still more, since I had been brought up among girls with a noticeable tendency to babble.

The party, as a result of the martinis, followed by much wine and port, picked up steam. One group, including George and the Baron's daughter, embarked on a boating expedition on the baronial lake. The boat sank, which added to the party spirit. Emboldened by port, I inveigled Tish into the rose garden and kissed her, a gesture which she returned with gratifying warmth. Unfortunately, the Premier Baroness caught us *in flagrante,* to everyone's embarrassment.

Later, I learned that the Premier Baroness had that very night written a letter to Mrs. Hankey, Tish's mother, who was living in London, recounting the episode in the rose garden and warning in strong terms of the dangers inherent in Tish's "hot Spanish blood." Tish, it turned out, had been brought up in Gibraltar, where her grandfather, an English knight, had married a beautiful Spanish girl. The beautiful Spanish girl produced several beautiful half-Spanish girls, including Tish's mother, who married Arthur Hankey, an Etonian younger son, and produced Tish and Ian. I never met Ian. He was in the King's Royal Rifle Corps too, but before I was sent to Africa he was killed in the desert in 1942, age nineteen.

I also later discovered something else—that Tish, despite the lipstick and the martinis, was only sixteen when I met

59

her. Even so, that night in the rose garden I had fallen in love with her, and though she has always denied it, I still think she had fallen in love with me. We were married two years later, just after D-Day, in a Catholic chapel in London. A buzz bomb above us ran out of gas as we were saying the marriage vows.

I NEVER DID get to know the other sick people in the leukemia ward on more than a nodding basis. Most of us spent most of our time in bed. Wandering occasionally in the corridors, trundling our I.V.s in front of us, we would pass each other and nod and smile with an effort.

Sometimes there would be a sad little group gathered, untalkatively, in front of the television set in the recreation room. It was usually possible to tell at a glance from the color of their skin which of them were undergoing chemotherapy or had just completed it and were "in remission." The patients in the laminar flow rooms never left their rooms and were of course invisible, except for an occasional glimpse from the corridor, when a door was open.

Aside from Tish, I had plenty of company. There was a telephone in my room, and there were a good many calls outgoing and incoming, including one from President Nixon. The President is not very good at small talk, and neither am I, so it was not a very profound or lengthy conversation. He remarked that he hoped to visit me at NIH. I could hardly say so, but I rather hoped he wouldn't. Emmet Hughes had recently denounced me in the *New York Times Magazine* as a mere Presidential toady, his chief evidence being that

I saw Henry Kissinger quite often and that I failed to echo the approved liberal line on Vietnam. A Presidential visit would be taken as proof of the charge. More important, since neither of us is good at small talk, and I would be lying in bed hooked up to an I.V., a visit from the President would be sure to be an embarrassing occasion.

The President, fortunately, never came, but I had a lot of other visitors. Joe and Susan Mary came most days, and there were almost always two or three other people at our picnic lunches. We would move into the recreation room and drink martinis and eat sandwiches supplied by Tish or Susan Mary. Quite often we achieved a certain gaiety. Once the gaiety was shattered. A pretty girl rushed through the room and into the bathroom, and we could hear her sobbing wildly. Her mother was in a laminar flow room and had just died.

Our picnics got us in trouble with a head nurse. Joe came in one day, ostentatiously waving a bottle of Scotch, and she sharply reprimanded him. "This is a federal reservation," she said. "No liquor is allowed." We mumbled something, hid our glasses, and went on drinking.

Later, I got into still deeper trouble with her. John Glick had prescribed a couple of bowel-softening pills per day. This was because of my low platelets; he wanted no trouble from internal bleeding. Then, when I complained of constipation, he gave me a very powerful laxative. After I had exploded for a couple of hours, the head nurse came in with my bowel pills. I remarked mildly that under the circumstances I hardly needed them.

"I'll put you down as refused," she said furiously, in the manner of the Red Queen sentencing a Knight. We were enemies; I thought of her as "the battle ax," and "the sergeant major," and I'm sure she thought of me in equally uncomplimentary terms. But by the time I had left NIH, she had become my favorite nurse. She knew her business, and when you are in fear of death a nurse who knows her business is a pearl beyond price. I also discovered that behind the sergeant major's manner there was a kind and nice woman.

Some kind of routine or discipline is, moreover, necessary in a hospital (although, just in case, I got John Glick to promise to prescribe a martini before lunch and two before dinner, if I was put in the laminar flow room). Sometimes the routine is carried to ridiculous extremes.

One morning, about a week after I'd been hospitalized, after a bad night (it's hard to sleep if you're afraid) a cheerful young nurse shook me awake at 6 A.M. to weigh me. "For Chrissakes, can't you weigh me just as well in an hour or so?" I asked. She was embarrassed, and it wasn't her fault. So I wearily got out of bed and stepped on the machine.

Most of the nurses were remarkably nice and long-suffering, and they made an almost excessive effort to be cheerful. Some of them did not appreciate my feeble attempts at humor, though.

There was, for example, one all-business nurse who presided over one of the more esoteric tests John Glick ordered for me. In this test, which is designed to search out any hidden malignancy, you are given a shot of radio-active isotopes, and a huge X-ray machine then passes over your body, starting at the head, while a ghostly image of your body is reproduced on a sort of television screen. My head appeared first, and my nose, which like that of all Alsops of my generation is very large, wholly dominated the screen.

I had been reading too much P. G. Wodehouse. "No

doubt you have noted, nurse," I said, "the aquiline and aristocratic cast of my features."

She looked at me, then at the screen. "Looks just like any other ordinary patient," she said starchily.

Polly Wisner and Clayton Fritchey, both old friends, came in for a picnic lunch after I'd had the test, and I told this small, not very funny story. They both laughed, and then Polly made quickly for the bathroom. I think she was afraid she was going to cry, and maybe she did. Any humor in 13E has a certain gallows quality, even very feeble imitation-Wodehouse humor.

I spent a lot of my time reading—nothing very profound, since I was in a mood for escape, not profundity. When I had had enough of Wodehouse and Trollope I turned to *The Day of the Jackal,* the best seller about an attempted assassination of de Gaulle. I was enjoying it thoroughly when one of the characters told another that his girl friend had "luke-something." I closed the book hurriedly, sure that the girl friend would soon die. In fact, I'm told, she didn't, but I've never finished the novel.

When I wasn't reading for escape, I spent a lot of time trying to remember quotations. I have a small store of familiar quotations and Latin tags in my head, mostly from school and college days, and I almost always get them wrong. I have, in Byron's phrase, "just enough of learning to misquote."

For example, I kept trying to remember T. S. Eliot's eternal Footman. After much brain cudgeling, I scribbled in my notebook:

> I have seen the moment of my greatness flicker.
> I have seen the eternal Footman hold my coat,
>   and snicker.
> In short, I was afraid.

Looking it up later, I found I had it wrong, as usual—Eliot had put a comma after "snicker," and prefaced the next line with an "And" to make a single sentence. I have a feeling my version is punchier.

Then there were snatches of nonsense verse, for which I've always had a fondness. From Belloc's *Cautionary Tales*:

> The chief defect of Henry King
> Was chewing little bits of string.
> At last he swallowed some which tied
> Itself in ugly knots inside.
> Physicians of the utmost fame
> Were called at once; but when they came
> They answered, as they took their fees,
> "There is no cure for this disease."

And an old favorite by Clarence Day (I thought it was by James Thurber and remembered it all wrong, but my brother John, who has a much better memory than I, set me right):

> Farewell, my friends—
> Farewell and hail!
> I'm off to seek the Holy Grail.
>   I cannot tell you why.
> Remember, please, when I am gone,
> 'Twas Aspiration led me on.
> Tiddlely-widdlely tootle-oo,
> All I want is to stay with you,
>   But here I go. Good-bye.

The thrust of these snippets of memory suggests a melancholy frame of mind, but I found it oddly comforting to dig into my small store of remembered quotations. It was a way of papering over misery. I always liked the story about Winston Churchill as a subaltern in the Boer War when he had to spend a couple of days hiding from the Boers in a dark hole. He passed the time quite happily reciting to himself all the familiar quotations and Latin tags he could recall. This is at least a better way to spend the time than fearing death.

I also found amusing and oddly comforting a note which arrived with a very pretty flower from Alice Longworth—Cousin Alice, as I've called her for more than forty years. (She is my first cousin, once removed.) It was scribbled on a yellowed calling card—the card looked as though it dated from the twenties—and it read: "Stew—what a nuisance—love from your aged coz."

Acute leukemia—a nuisance? The note is a nice example of Mrs. Longworth's highly idiosyncratic style, which shapes her rather macabre humor. She has had two mastectomies and likes to refer to herself, preferably before the most easily shockable audience, as "Washington's topless octogenarian." She also likes to call herself "Washington's only perambulatory monument."

My favorite Longworthism is her admonition: "Never trust a man who parts his hair under his left armpit." The warning is valid. Those who try to cover their bald spots by growing their hair long and combing it sideways (General Douglas MacArthur, for example, or Senator Arthur Vandenberg) are providing solid evidence of an abnormal vanity. Abnormally vain people have no sense of humor about themselves, and they thus lack balance and are not to be trusted.

The day after Mrs. Longworth's flower arrived, Susan Mary, my charming sister-in-law, paid a visit while Joe was tied up on some journalistic chore. She had bad news. Tommy Thompson—Llewellyn Thompson, twice Ambassador to Moscow and a very old friend—had entered Georgetown Hospital the day before I had. His ulcer had been bothering

66

him again. The doctors, Susan Mary said, had opened him up, found an inoperable cancer, and closed him up again.

Tish and I had seen him only a few nights before, when we were both in Georgetown Hospital. It was the evening of the day when Dr. Perry told me I had AML. We had taken an elevator to the roof, where you can eat cafeteria food outdoors. I was in a bathrobe, picking unhappily at a chilly bacon-lettuce-and-tomato sandwich, when Tommy came wandering up, also in a bathrobe. We chatted for a bit, and then he drifted off. Tish and I said nothing about my diagnosis; it seemed pointless. I wonder if Tommy knew, or suspected, what was wrong with him and also said nothing.

There were times when I was able to forget that I too had an inoperable cancer. But there were also times, like that moment of fear in the auditorium on the fourteenth floor, when the inescapable reality suddenly overcame me. One such time came in early August, a few days before I was sent home from NIH. Dr. Edward Henderson, chief of the leukemia section and John Glick's boss, had come into my room for a talk. He is a shy man, rather dour-faced, in his thirties. He lacks a warm bedside manner, but his obvious intelligence and competence are more encouraging to a sick man than any bedside manner.

We chatted for a while about me (one of the compensations for being hospitalized with a serious but puzzling disease is that everybody talks about you). He described how atypical my disease was in several ways, and then I asked a question which had been on my mind for several days.

"Is there any chance I have aplastic anemia?" I asked. Aplastic anemia is a serious marrow disease, but it is not malignant.

Dr. Henderson hesitated for a moment. "No," he said.

"Then I do have some form of cancer, AML or something else?"

"Yes," he said quietly.

He left, and I started writing a note of thanks to Kay Halle, for a book she had sent me. Kay was a close friend of Randolph Churchill, who was also a friend of mine. She stayed often at Chartwell, the Churchill country place, and she has edited two books about Winston Churchill and one about Randolph.

I wrote my letter as a takeoff on Winston's famous speech of defiance. "We will fight amongst the platelets," I wrote. "We will fight in the bone marrow. We will fight in the peripheral blood. We will never surrender."

Having written this, I began, for the first time in about fifty years, to cry. I was utterly astonished, and also dismayed. I was brought up to believe that for a man to weep in public is the ultimate indignity, a proof of unmanliness. Only my elderly roommate was in the room, and he hadn't noticed. I ducked into our tiny shared bathroom, and closed the door, and sat down on the toilet, and turned on the bath water, so that nobody could hear me, and cried my heart out. Then I dried my eyes on the toilet paper and felt a good deal better.

I suppose this sudden unmanliness resulted from the combination of Dr. Henderson's monosyllables and Churchill. When Dr. Henderson said "no" to my first question and "yes" to my second, a small light went out, a light of hope that I might not have cancer after all.

As for Churchill, of all the public figures I have known, he is my only enduring hero. (I have had stirrings of hero worship for Franklin Roosevelt, John F. Kennedy, and Robert McNamara, but they have dimmed with time.) Perhaps

68

an incurable Anglophilia influenced my admiration for Churchill, and perhaps also a nostalgia for a time that has passed and will never come again—wartime London, wonderful parties at Rosa Lewis's Cavendish Hotel, falling in love with Tish. But there are also, surely, less subjective reasons for admiring the great old man—his courage, his humor, his style. What impressed me most, oddly enough, was his genius for recognizing the obvious. (I think, but am not sure, that the phrase was his own.)

He displayed that genius when he recognized that Hitler really did intend to conquer Europe, a notion poohpoohed by almost all fashionable and intelligent people in the thirties. In my own view, he displayed this special genius even more clearly in the series of speeches he made in the late forties and early fifties, when he was supposedly in decline.

In those speeches (which should rank, I think, with his wartime speeches) he examined in its every aspect the essential problem facing the Western nations—the problem of living in the same world both with Soviet-style communism and with the nuclear weapon. By a process of recognizing the obvious, he reached the conclusion that the nuclear weapon, in its very horror, might offer both sides of the divided world a long period of peace, "a peace of mutual terror." But he insisted on the essential condition, that the terror be truly mutual. Churchill's peace of mutual terror is the peace we have been living with all these years, and it is at least very much better than a nuclear war. But his condition remains essential.

I met Mr. Churchill (as he was then) only once, but that occasion remains vivid in my memory. (The recollection, it must be admitted, has been refurbished by a good many journalistic retellings.) It was in the summer of 1950.

69

I was on a reporting tour of Europe, for the column I wrote with Joe for the now defunct Herald Tribune Syndicate. In Rome I ran into Randolph Churchill, the great man's son, who was writing pieces (when he was sober and the mood was upon him) for the Beaverbrook press.

Randolph and I decided to have a look at Soviet-occupied Austria by train, via Florence and Trieste. We were joined on the train by Culbert Olson, who had been a Democratic populist governor of California during the thirties. He was a tall handsome man of about seventy, with a flat midwestern accent and a hyena laugh when he thought something funny.

Randolph insisted that we stop in Florence, to inspect "the ancient glories of this great city" and also to renew his acquaintance with Mrs. Violet Trefusis, who had a villa outside the town. Violet Trefusis, Randolph explained, was known as "Mrs. Trefusis, Never Refusis." She was the daughter of the famous Mrs. Keppel, who had decidedly not refused Edward VII, and she was thought to have royal blood flowing in her veins. She turned out to be a woman of a certain age and great charm, which she exercised with startling effect on Governor Olson, who fell briefly but passionately in love with her. I do not know whether she lived up to her name.

We had a bibulous dinner in Florence (every dinner with Randolph tended to be bibulous), and then we set forth to view the "ancient glories." Randolph and the Governor staged a fine scene.

"Know what I'd do, if I was governor here?" the Governor asked, in his flat nasal twang, as he viewed the twilit splendors of the Duomo. "I'd tear the whole place down."

"*What?*" roared Randolph.

"Yessir," said the Governor. "Tear the whole place

70

down. Lay down a modern sewage system. Build some good modern public housing. Then you'd have a city fit for people to live in."

"TEAR FLORENCE DOWN?" howled Randolph. "Destroy this ancient monument of Western civilization? Replace the gilded splendors of this great city with public housing?"

"Yessir," said Governor Olson. "I'd tear the whole goddam place down." Then he cackled his hyena laugh, driving Randolph to paroxysms of eloquent fury. It was a great show, a classic Anglo-American vaudeville performance. We were joined by a crowd of ragged Italian kids, who hooted at the mad Englishman and the crazy American, and the show lasted for the better part of an hour.

Governor Olson fell in love again in Trieste and left us. Randolph and I pushed on into Soviet-occupied Austria, where Randolph almost got me thrown in jail by the Soviet police, but that is another story. By the time we parted, we were friends. Randolph was not an easy man to be friends with. When drunk, which was quite often, he could be wholly intolerable. And yet he was a man of great qualities —intelligence, courage, and a certain unexpected sweetness. Above all, it never occurred to him to be anything but himself—except very rarely, when he foolishly tried to be Winston Churchill. He reminded me, in a way, of my cousin Ted Roosevelt, the President's son and Alice Longworth's brother, who was my boss and friend when I worked at Doubleday Doran as a junior editor before the war. There were great differences, of course, but Ted was also a man of intelligence, courage, and unexpected sweetness, and he too bore the burden of being the son of a great man. Ted died on the Normandy beachhead, and Randolph died in 1968. For both of them I still feel a deep affection.

71

When I got to London a week or so after we parted in Austria, Randolph called me at my hotel and invited me to lunch at Chartwell the next day. I naturally supposed that there would be a large number of interesting and important people at the luncheon, and that I could perform the function of a fly on the wall.

Instead, the lunch party consisted of the old man, Randolph, and myself, and at first it was a most uncomfortable affair. Mr. Churchill was dressed in a siren suit and looked like an angry old baby. He responded to my shy greetings with an angry harrumphing noise. I think Randolph had sprung me on him at the last moment, and that I was not at all a welcome addition.

We had no cocktail, not even a glass of sherry. The first course was a delicious soup, which we ate in near-total silence, interrupted only by an occasional harrumph or slurping noise. Randolph was clearly almost as nervous as I was. With the second course—fish, if I remember correctly—a bottle of excellent champagne was served; Mr. Churchill and I consumed it between us, since Randolph was officially on the wagon. Then there was another bottle of champagne. The effect of the champagne on Mr. Churchill was like that of the morning sun on an opening flower.

He began to talk, through the champagne, and then through port and a small bottle of a special cognac, which he consumed alone, since the champagne and the port were almost too much for me. He was talking, I suppose, for his own amusement—I was a thirty-six-year-old American journalist, of whom he had probably never heard, and there was no good reason to waste such talk on me. For the talk was good, very good, wise and witty and malicious by turns.

I remember only snatches of it. I remember saying something about a member of the Attlee labor cabinet, whom I had interviewed the day before. Mr. Churchill's response was very much that of the grandson of the Duke of Marlborough.

"I wouldn't have him for a gardener," he said. He paused for a moment of consideration. "I wouldn't have him for an *under*gardener."

I think it was Randolph who introduced the name of Anthony Eden into the conversation. Churchill was leader of His Majesty's opposition at the time, and Eden was his number two, as he had been for years and would remain for still more years.

"Ah, yes, Anthony," he said. "Dear Anthony. When there is a debate scheduled in which I do not greatly wish to take part—about sewer systems or the like—I telephone Anthony. I tell him, 'This is a great opportunity for you, my boy, an opportunity for you to make a great name for yourself. *You can lead the debate.*'" The old man smiled the smile of a naughty, happy child.

At one point, I remember, he pulled a crumpled newspaper clipping out of his pocket and read it aloud. It was part of an interview with Bernard Baruch, who had said something to the effect that he greatly admired his old friend Winston Churchill but that unfortunately Churchill knew nothing whatever about economics. After reading the clipping, Mr. Churchill treated us to a pyrotechnical but totally incomprehensible disquisition on the global economic situation. He was not without vanity.

Toward the end of the luncheon, vaguely aware that I was an American, he began to talk about his wartime relationship with Franklin Roosevelt and then about America in general. He made a ringing rhetorical tribute to "your great country" and concluded with a peroration in ripe Churchillian style.

"America," he said musingly. "America. A great and

powerful country. Like some strong horse pulling the rest of the world up behind it out of the slough of despond, towards peace and prosperity."

Then he fixed his old blue eyes on me accusingly.

"But will America stay the course?" he asked.

I said rather weakly that I was sure it would, and Mr. Churchill led the way outdoors. He led us first to a rather muddy small pool. A secret service man, who had obviously been through the routine before, produced a tobacco tin filled with grubs, and Mr. Churchill began to drop the grubs in the water. Instantly, a number of large fat goldfish appeared.

"See that one?" Mr. Churchill said. "Worth fully four pounds, I daresay. I paid only ten shillings for him." He pointed out several other fish, estimating with satisfaction his profit on each. Then he led us to a series of small waterways, which led down to a much larger pool.

"This will surprise you, my boy," he said, and turned a spigot. I was indeed surprised, for the water—was it that last glass of port?—seemed to flow uphill.

The old man stumped down toward the larger pool. In the middle was what appeared to be a bicycle tire, with mirrors attached to its rim. Mr. Churchill pressed a button, and the tire began slowly to revolve. The contraption, he said proudly, was his own invention. The mirrors reflected the rays of the sun, thus frightening off the marauding birds that stole the fish out of his pool. Just as he finished his explanation, it began to rain.

"Unfortunately for my invention," said Mr. Churchill, his tone bordering on the tragic, "on this small island, the sun hardly ever shines."

Mr. Churchill gave us a guided tour of his painting studio and proudly displayed a handsome brick wall he had

74

built. When I left, late in the afternoon, he was using another of his inventions, a peculiar contraption of counterweights and pulleys with which he was attempting, unsuccessfully, to uproot a small tree.

Throughout, he displayed a kind of childishness—there is no other word for it. His pride in his dubious knowledge of economics or his inventions was completely unfeigned, like a child's. He was what Mark Twain once called Andrew Carnegie, "the human being unconcealed." The carapace or outer tegument which people grow to protect and conceal themselves from other people had somehow never grown on him. This was, perhaps, one secret of his enormous charm. He was the most undisappointing public man I have ever met.

As for that question he asked me, that was the era of American confidence, and it never occurred to me that America might not "stay the course." I am not quite so sure now. But at least one other thing the old man said at the lunch table has proved right so far.

He had been talking about Hitler and the "Naazis," and then he began to survey the then current scene. Stalin's blockade of Berlin had been broken, and so had the Soviet attempt to capture Greece, thanks largely to Harry Truman's "Greek-Turkish aid." But the Korean war had just started, and the international horizon, as discerned by Mr. Churchill, was very dark.

"And yet, you know," he said, "as soon as Hitler took power, I *knew* a great world war was coming. I felt war in my bones. But I do not think a great world war is coming now. I do not feel war in my bones."

That was more than two decades ago, and the feeling in Mr. Churchill's bones has so far proved accurate. Indeed, as of this writing, a third world war seems a lot less likely than it did in 1950. The essential reason is, I suppose, that so far the terror has continued to be mutual. It begins to seem at least possible, bar madness or miscalculation, that the "peace of mutual terror" will prevail, even unto the third and fourth generation.

At any rate, after I had wept in the bathroom that day on the thirteenth floor of NIH, I consoled myself with the thought that Mr. Churchill used to weep, when he was moved, quite publicly and shamelessly.

DURING THOSE FIRST two weeks in NIH—from July 21 to August 6, 1971—I lived on two levels. One level concerned what was going on in my mind. The other level concerned what was going on in my body, and more especially in my marrow and my blood. The second level turned out to be a lot more puzzling and mysterious than the first.

A great debate, John Glick explained to me, started in Georgetown about my diagnosis, and it raged on at NIH. After John Glick gave me my first blood transfusion, my energy and my reportorial instincts revived, and I found myself taking an increasing part in the debate. A couple of pages after the scribble "leukemia," I find in my notebook another scribble: "This is a most interesting experience, although one wishes one were not so personally involved."

The experience was interesting partly because my disease was unusual. It refused to behave like classic AML—although AML remained the official diagnosis—or like any other conventional form of marrow cancer. I think I can claim to be the first to state categorically that AML could not be the correct diagnosis of what was wrong with me.

Perhaps because my case was so peculiar, I had a good many visits from doctors on the NIH staff. Three or four times a day, one doctor or another (I never did get all their names straight) would wander in, to ask me questions and chat. One of these doctors, a rather pompous middle-aged man, began talking about the characteristics common to people who had AML. Most Orientals, Chinese and Japanese especially, he said, seemed virtually immune to the disease.

"This of course isn't a scientific observation," said the doctor. "It's just an impression. But my impression is that AML is largely a disease of white middle-class or lower-middle-class people of rather limited intelligence."

To be placed in such a category outraged me. "Goddammit, doctor," I said, and I was only half joking, "I can't *possibly* have AML."

John Glick and the other NIH specialists were themselves increasingly of his opinion, though on more scientific and less snobbish grounds. In the beginning most of the specialists, after peering at my marrow slides, agreed that I probably had some peculiar form of AML. But Dr. Harvey Gralnick, the chief morphologist, disagreed. He suspected that I had some atypical form of dysproteinemia, a marrow cancer but not a leukemia.

Dysproteinemia, John Glick told me, had a somewhat longer average survival time than AML, and the chemotherapy was milder. There was also a minority view that I might have some unusual form of Hodgkin's disease, or a related lymphatic disorder. This would be good news, since Hodgkin's disease in some forms is actually curable, if caught early enough.

I find a cryptic note in my notebook: "Imagine hoping you have Hodgkin's disease."

After my temperature had subsided and I began to feel reasonably well, I enjoyed talking with John and the other doctors, the more so because the conversations were all about me. On Thursdays, a whole platoon of doctors, eight to fifteen at a time, led by Dr. Henderson, would troop through the ward. There were always some visiting doctors, often foreigners, and since my case was peculiar they would spend a good deal of time crowded around my bed. Being a talkative fellow, I would take my part in these conversations—sometimes a bit more than my part. John Glick and I had taken to referring to me as "Dr. Alsop." One morning, he introduced me to the visiting platoon as "Doctor Alsop." He was embarrassed, and I was amused, but nobody noticed.

The debate about my peculiar disease intensified after someone remembered and unearthed the marrow slides of Mrs. Y. The case of Mrs. Y had John Glick as tensely fascinated as a Sherlock Holmes confronted by the Case of the Speckled Band. As a matter of fact John Glick looks a bit like Sherlock Holmes—or would, with a deerstalker, a cloak and a pipe.

Mrs. Y was a housewife who was diagnosed as having AML and given chemotherapy for that disease. The diagnosis, it turned out later, was incorrect. She had, instead of AML, an atypical form of dysproteinemia. She died three and a half years after her chemotherapy, of pneumonia. She might have been saved if she had been treated immediately with antibiotics, but she was a gay and rather feckless lady, and she didn't report to NIH until it was too late.

Somebody in the hematology department remembered Mrs. Y's marrow and dug it out of the files. It looked almost exactly like my marrow, a fact which seemed to support Dr. Gralnick's theory that I too had an atypical dysproteinemia. Like me, she had about 40 percent abnormal cells, and like me she was hypocellular, meaning she had few cells of any sort, good or bad. John Glick labeled my marrow slide Alsop and hers Y and then transposed the names. None of the specialists could tell for certain which was which.

I find another note in my notebook: "Every little helps. If Mrs. Y lasted three and a half years, then I might too, and that at least is beating the odds."

A man with an inoperable cancer clutches at straws. Toward the end of the first week, Amanda called and said that Tom Joyce, an able reporter in the *Newsweek* Washington bureau, had been diagnosed as a leukemic, and he was fine now. Hope springs eternal. I called Tom and asked him about the diagnosis. It turned out that when he was reporting in Vietnam for the *Detroit News*, he had suddenly been taken very ill. He was flown home, and tests showed that his blood was in bad shape. He was sent to NIH and had a bone marrow. The marrow was clean. The doctors finally found out what was wrong. He had a parasite nibbling away at his liver. It was the same sort of parasite that killed poor Marguerite Higgins. In the end, Tom shook it off. No hopeful parallel with the case of S. Alsop, of course.

After this disappointment, Ed Henderson came in with John Glick, and we had a long talk—about, as usual, me. Henderson dwelt on my "pancytopenia." He described how few cells of any sort, normal or abnormal, I had in my marrow.

"It sounds to me," I said, "like the end of some great battle, in which the slaughter has been intense, and both sides are so exhausted that all fighting has stopped."

"No," said Dr. Henderson. "The battle is still going on."

It is a curious feeling to have the inside of your bones

a battlefield. I amused myself by trying to think of military analogies. Antietam? Gettysburg? The victory of Pyrrhus over the Romans at Asculum? ("One more such victory and I am lost.") Perhaps, for that matter, Vietnam, for both sides the most unwinnable war in modern history.

John gave me several marrow tests—more than would have been necessary if I had had a classic, easily identifiable case of leukemia—and one biopsy. The biopsy meant getting a bigger hunk of me, for more detailed observation. This is done with an instrument that looks like a miniature pair of sharp sugar tongs. I have unusually hard bones, and John twisted two of these small instruments all out of shape before he finally got into the bone.

A marrow test is an unpleasant experience, and a biopsy is more so. But neither is nearly so unpleasant as waiting for the results. Every time I had a marrow test, there would be that hour or so of suspense, filled with the fear of a "fulmination" of the abnormal cells. The fulmination would be followed by chemotherapy, the laminar flow room, and the near certainty of death in a year or two.

But the abnormal cells (Thank you God, thank you Mother, thank you Father, thank you Aggie) did not fulminate. Instead, the percentage dropped off a bit, from 44 percent by the Georgetown count, to 40 percent, then to 38 percent. Above all, there were no "blasts in the peripheral blood"—the abnormal cells were found only in the bone marrow. This, as John Glick explained to me, gave him leeway, room to turn around. If I had had a lot of blasts in the peripheral blood, he would have had no choice but to put me into chemotherapy right away. Otherwise, the blasts in the blood would have eaten away at the blood, crowding out the life-giving good cells, and they would thus have ensured death in a matter of weeks at the most.

81

So the absence of blasts in the blood was good news, very good news indeed. But John added with characteristic candor that "those weirdos, the bad cells in your marrow—they look ugly, *really* ugly."

I find another note in my notebook, written after the biopsy:

"Maybe I am not lucky my case is so peculiar. Maybe I am very unlucky. Maybe it would have been better if I had had a classic AML, and I had been put into chemotherapy right away, before I knew what had happened to me. I would surely have died, but sometimes this suspense is hardly bearable."

This unhappy scribble bears on a question which obviously concerned John Glick deeply: how much to tell a cancer patient. He talked about it often. He told me that there are leukemia specialists known as "nihilists" who believe that AML patients, since they are virtually certain to die anyway, should be told nothing whatever about their disease and be left to die without chemotherapy. (As chemotherapy has improved, this school has become increasingly rare.) According to this school, a person newly diagnosed as an acute leukemic should be told only that he has anemia, and given occasional hemoglobin and platelet transfusions to keep him going until the time inevitably comes—almost always in less than four months—when he will die of infection, for lack of granulocytes to protect him.

Sir William Osler, the great nineteenth-century physician, once remarked that to die of a fever was as good a way to die as any, and an acute leukemic, if he is not kept alive with antibiotics, usually dies of infection very quickly. Meanwhile, having been told only that he is anemic and that the anemia is being treated, he is not hopelessly unhappy. To be hopeless is to be unhappy, and the AML patient who is told the truth is hopeless and therefore unnecessarily unhappy. So runs the argument of the nihilists.

Many doctors, John Glick told me, half accept this argument. "In a good many hospitals," he said, "treatment of AML is halfhearted and unaggressive, since in any case the patient is sure to die." John made this remark during my first week at NIH and it was a bit hard to take, since at that time my official diagnosis was still AML. The remark was typical of NIH policy, as exemplified by those Rules of Admission I had come across on the fourteenth floor. NIH policy calls for (1) aggressive treatment, right up to the patient's last breath, and (2) complete candor with the patient.

No doubt there is a lot to be said for this NIH policy. If the patient knows as much as possible about his disease, he can sometimes help the doctor with his case. For example, I came up with "Dr. Alsop's theory" to explain my sudden fever, and Dr. Glick thought it was probably a valid theory.

On the Thursday before I was hospitalized, I went wading in the upper Potomac with Sandy Sanderson of the Maryland Fish and Wildlife Service. I had read a piece by Sandy in *Maryland Magazine* about bass fishing in the Potomac. I'd written to him to find out more, and he had kindly offered to take me fly fishing for small-mouth bass in the upper Potomac, near Needwood.

We'd spent several hours wading waist deep in the river, dragging Sandy's boat behind us, on a rope tied to our belts. We saw some very big bass jumping, but they flatly refused to take the fly. I'd felt a bit pooped—not surprisingly, since my hemoglobin count must have been well under 8.

I had a small unhealed cut on my knee, presumably a result of my peculiar habit of hitting myself with my racket

83

when I serve, though the cut was higher than usual. Dr. Alsop's theory was that the cut had been infected by the waters of the Potomac, by no means unpolluted even in its upper reaches. Dr. Glick thought Dr. Alsop might have hit on the right answer. There was no way of knowing, though. The cut looked a bit red and ugly, but there was no visible infection. The pus which makes an infection visible was absent—pus consists of granulocytes, and I hadn't enough of them to make any visible display.

At NIH, saving the individual patient is not the essential mission. Enormous efforts are made to do so, or at least to prolong the patient's life to the last possible moment. But the basic purpose is not to save that particular patient's life but to find means of saving the lives of others, in other hospitals in this country and throughout the world. In this sense, although the NIH doctors hate the phrase, the leukemic patients are guinea pigs, and the emotions of the guinea pigs are not the first consideration. (I have been proud of being, so far, so unusual and instructive a guinea pig; presumably the government made a good investment in my case.)

My own view on this matter falls somewhere between the nihilists and the NIH view. A patient should be told the truth, and nothing but the truth—but not the whole truth. I find scribbled in my notebook, after the notes about the placard in the auditorium: "A man who must die will die more easily if he is left a little spark of hope that he may not die after all. My rule would be: Never tell a victim of terminal cancer the whole truth—tell him that he *may* die, even that he will *probably* die, but do not tell him that he *will* die."

I gather that John Glick disagrees with me; he believes in the truth, the whole truth, and nothing but the truth. It was certainly instructive to have so candid a mentor, and it may have been useful to him too, in making up his mind about my case. But it was not an experience without pain.*

On August 6, seventeen days after I entered NIH, Ed Henderson and John made up their minds about my case. My diagnosis was no longer officially AML, John Glick told me, although most of the doctors still believed I had some peculiar and idiosyncratic form of AML. The main reason they so believed was that about 75 percent of the abnormal cells in my marrow looked like "myeloblasts," the malignant cells that attack the marrow in AML.

But in other ways my symptoms were wholly uncharacteristic. If I had a classic AML, my marrow would be chock full of leukemic cells, and I would probably have other symptoms I didn't have—bleeding from the gums, for example, a fullness in the belly resulting from enlarged liver or spleen, bone pain from the excess of malignant cells in the marrow, and above all myeloblasts, or malignant cells, in the blood. As long as there were no blasts in the blood, there was no rush to treat me.

Because my symptoms were so uncharacteristic, John Glick decided on this diagnosis: "Pancytopenia of unknown etiology." Translated from the medicalese, this means, "This patient has damn few cells, normal or abnormal, but we don't know why."

They decided to do nothing—to send me home without treatment. They would be keeping an eye on me, John Glick said. I'd be having a blood test every week, probably

---

* John Glick, reading this paragraph, reminds me that when I was admitted to NIH he was almost as much a new boy as I was—he had only been there two or three weeks. After two years of experience in treating cancer patients at NIH, he still believes in telling a patient the basic facts of his situation. But he says, "I am much less clinical," and he agrees in substance with the note I scribbled in my notebook after seeing the placard in the auditorium.

85

a marrow test every other week. He gave me his home and office numbers and told me to call him right away if my temperature went over 100 or if I had a chill, unusual pain anywhere, an atypical cough, fast or painful urine, an earache, sore throat.

He was, he said, especially worried about infection, because my granulocyte count was so low. "I'd be a lot happier if we could get your granulocytes up over five hundred, and happier still if we could get them over a thousand. But there are more sources of infection here in the hospital than there are in your own house, so there's no reason not to send you home."

I asked him what was his best guess about what would happen to me, and he said that he just didn't know.

"We'll just wait for the nature of the disease to declare itself." He paused for a moment, thoughtfully. "I don't want to mislead you. It is possible—just barely possible—that whatever you have will go away, that you'll have a spontaneous remission. But in this kind of disease spontaneous remissions are very, very rare. It's a lot more likely that when the disease declares itself we will put you into chemotherapy to induce a remission."

"And after you've induced a remission, I'm statistically certain to have a relapse. Right? The bad cells are totally certain to come back?"

"Almost totally," said John Glick.

"Why? Why do they come back?"

"If we knew that," he said, "we'd know what caused them in the first place—we'd know what caused the cancer, therefore we'd be on the track of a cure. Whoever answers your question is a certain winner of the Nobel prize."

O N AUGUST 6 Tish fetched me at NIH
and drove me home. Home is a large, rather ugly house in
Cleveland Park. Fortunately, except in rush hour, it's only
about twenty minutes from the NIH complex in Bethesda.
The house is set in over an acre of woods, with a tennis
court carved out of the side of a hill. We bought the place
in 1950, when our Georgetown house became too small
for our expanding family.

The house is comfortable, and I have enjoyed myself
in it often, for more than twenty years, but I have no feeling
for it as a house. It reminds me of Winston Churchill's remark, as recounted in Harold Macmillan's memoirs. A waiter
set before Churchill a large and tasteless pudding. "Waiter,"
Churchill said, "pray remove this pudding. It has no theme."

Our Washington house has no theme. It has no character, no interesting or individual quality. The central part
was the caretaker's house for what was once a big farm—
the original farmhouse, a handsome antebellum dark-red
brick house, is just visible from our porch when the leaves
are off the trees. A dining room wing and a living room wing
were built during the 1930s. The result is roomy and con-
venient, but characterless. When Phil Watts and my brother

John and I talked about selling the house in anticipation of my death, the thought of doing so aroused no painful sentiments, while the thought of selling Needwood Forest was almost as painful as the notion of selling my daughter, Elizabeth, might have been.

There are some things in the house, though, that mean a good deal to me, or at least amuse me. We Alsops are thing-oriented—we all like objects, especially if we inherited them, and more especially if they are valuable. We like money too, though no Alsop has ever been really rich. There are unkind persons who maintain that money is our favorite, and often our only, subject of conversation.

Among the objects I inherited was a gravy boat with the letters REVERE cut into the bottom. To Tish and myself it looked like a Victorian object, and we used to leave it casually on the dining room sideboard. I assumed the REVERE was the mark of the Revere Copper and Brass Company, a Connecticut firm whose plant I remembered seeing years ago, when I took the train from Hartford to New York. Then an insurance assessor told me the sauce boat was an authentic product of "the patriot" ("One if by land, two if by sea") and that the last such piece had sold for $18,000. We hastily put the thing in a bank vault, and eventually we sold it, for a lot more than $18,000, since it was doing us no good in the bank and there were plenty of things, including a tennis court, that we wanted much more than a rather ugly silver sauce boat.

Still on the dining room sideboard, and scattered elsewhere in the dining room, are various pieces of china with a peculiar oriental version of a federal eagle painted on them. Before I did my piece on the family for the *Saturday Evening Post,* my attitude toward these bits of china—sauceboats, teapots, cups and saucers—was rather like that of Wordsworth's nonhero, Peter Bell, toward a primrose:

A primrose by a river's brim
A yellow primrose was to him,
And it was nothing more.

To me, the china was rather pretty china, and it was nothing more. But after I'd done the research for the *Post* piece, the china meant something more to me, for it told a good deal about the origins of the Alsop family. In the late eighteenth century and throughout the nineteenth, the Alsops lived in Middletown, Connecticut, in the early days one of New England's major ports. They made most of their money in the West Indies trade, shipping rum north and ice south. But they were also in the China trade, in a small way—hence the china, known variously as "export China" and "Chinese Lowestoft." American merchants in the China trade bought a lot of Chinese Lowestoft cheap.

The Alsops of that era were staunch federalists. The American eagle was the symbol of federalism—hence all those oriental-looking eagles on the export china. An early nineteenth-century Alsop, a poetaster called Richard, achieved some small measure of fame as a member of "the Hartford Wits" and is briefly mentioned in older editions of the *Encyclopedia Britannica*. He wrote a number of not at all witty poems worshiping "the great, immortal Washington" and "the illustrious Adams," and like all good federalists he had no use for Thomas Jefferson, whom he attacked in bad verse as a Jacobin, a dangerous revolutionary. His attitude toward Jefferson was precisely like that of my father toward Franklin Roosevelt, to whom Father frequently referred as "that crazy jack in the White House."

It surprised me to discover how consistently reactionary all my ancestors had been. One early Alsop, a rich New York merchant known in the family as "John, the nonsigner," attended the Continental Congress as a member of the New York delegation but refused to sign the Declaration of Independence, ostensibly on the grounds, as he wrote in his letter of resignation, that the Congress had closed the door to "reconciliation with Great Britain on just and honorable terms." One suspects that his real reason was that he was horrified by the text of the Declaration itself, drafted by that radical young fellow Thomas Jefferson—one can hear him muttering, "All men are created equal, indeed!"

An ancestor on my mother's side, one Peter Corne, was so uncompromising a Tory that he kept a life-size portrait of King George III in his cellar. Every evening, even after the Revolution, he would usher his large brood (including a great-great-grandmother of ours) down to the cellar by candlelight and command them, "Bow down to thy master."

Perhaps I am a federalist myself, and even a bit of a Tory. Before the Vietnam settlement, I got a letter from Anthony Lewis, the most dovish of the large collection of dove columnists on the *New York Times*. He wrote that "the last chance to save [the United States] from the eternal damnation that the Nazis earned Germany rests with conservatives like yourself."

The letter infuriated me, and with Tony Lewis's permission I quoted it and replied to it in an angry *Newsweek* piece. I was infuriated in part by the charge that Vietnam had earned this country "the eternal damnation that the Nazis earned Germany." In the very early days of the war I perceived, and wrote, that our commitment to Vietnam was based (to quote the title of a column of that period) on a "Great Miscalculation." But I did not and do not think that any of the foolish or brutal things we did in Vietnam was remotely comparable to Hitler's carefully planned and executed annihilation of six million Jews or his other manifold crimes against humanity.

I suspect that my fury was multiplied by Lewis's refer-

90

ence to "conservatives like yourself." I have always thought of myself as a liberal, and even a rather leftish liberal. The first piece I ever wrote and got paid for was published by *The Atlantic* before the Second World War—like most youthful efforts, it is a bit embarrassing to reread now. In it I proudly described myself as a "Marxist liberal."

It is true that in my Yale days I dabbled very superficially in Marxism. But what I really was—and I suppose I still am—was a rather conventional New Dealer. I much admired my distant cousin, Franklin Roosevelt, which irritated Father. He used to end dinner-table arguments about the New Deal and "that crazy jack in the White House" by suggesting that if I didn't like it here I could "go back to Russia." Since those days, I have voted for every Democratic Presidential candidate, including Hubert Humphrey in 1968, but decidedly not including George McGovern.

I suppose, by the standards of Tony Lewis and his kind of liberalism, this makes me a conservative. I think his kind of liberalism is disastrous, especially to the liberal interest. But then Father felt much the same way in the New Deal days.

Father's father, the third Joseph Alsop, was the lieutenant governor of Connecticut and aspired to the governorship. He died of a heart attack when he was presiding over an unseemly squabble in the state legislature—my brother John, an object lover like all Alsops, has the gavel he was banging futilely when the excitement became too much for him. Father, in his turn, desperately wanted to be governor. Being an old-fashioned Connecticut Yankee, he thought of the governorship of the sovereign state of Connecticut as the highest office in the land. When he was a young man, he was a leading Republican in the state senate, and he was thought to have had a good shot at the governorship.

Then Mother's Uncle Ted split the Republican Party

91

to run on the Progressive ticket for President in 1912. Father, a victim of the famous Roosevelt charm, headed the Progressive campaign organization and ran a hopeless race as a Progressive candidate for the Senate. That ended his gubernatorial hopes. In those days, regularity was the essential political virtue, and the regular Republican organization cast him into outer darkness. When we were children, there was occasional speculation in the Hartford papers about Father's running for governor, but nothing ever came of it. He never talked about it, but it was the one great disappointment of his life.

My younger brother John always wanted to be governor, too, and he came closer to making it than Father or Grandfather. In 1962 John won a bruising battle for the Republican gubernatorial nomination. He ran a good race, but 1962 was not a Republican year, and it didn't help a bit when John F. Kennedy, brother Joe's good friend and my semi-friend, campaigned for the Democratic ticket in Connecticut, where he was very popular. So John was the third Alsop to miss the grand gubernatorial prize.

When I was in my teens, my feelings about Pa, as we all called him, were ambivalent, and I think that was true of Joe and John too. Pa was a big man, well over six feet, with a big head and a long, authoritative nose. He always sat very much at the head of the table. He insisted on our dressing for dinner, and he would shout at us in company when we leaned back in the dining room chairs. (I shout at my children when they lean back in the same chairs, but it is the most I can do to get the boys to wear ties, sometimes, in the evening.) It is normal for teen-age boys to resist and on occasion to defy the domination of the male head of the family, but by the time Pa was an old man —he died at seventy-seven, which is old for an Alsop—I had great affection and admiration for him. He was *sui generis,* a Connecticut Yankee to his finger tips, and always very much his own man.

He was not at all a stuffy man. He took a month off in the winter to shoot quail, and another month in the summer to fish trout or salmon or play golf, and he enjoyed a good laugh, a couple of martinis before dinner, and a brandy afterward. But his political views seemed to his two older New Dealing sons (not to John, who was always a conservative by instinct) stuffy in the extreme. Once, after one of those dinner-table arguments, I asked Father a tactless question.

"Pa," I said, "How did you get to be such a reactionary?"

"GODDAMMIT, STEW," he roared in fury, "you don't seem to realize I was the leading Progressive in this state in 1912, and I'm just as much a Progressive today as I ever was. How can you say I'm a reactionary, you crazy jack?" He was genuinely angry at me. Maybe I was angry at Tony Lewis for similar reasons.

There is, I suppose, no escaping the genes. This is why I was relieved to discover that there was no blood relationship with the gentleman who was indirectly responsible for our dining room chairs; he was a relation by marriage. The chairs, vaguely Elizabethan in appearance, were carved in the Canary Islands during the First World War, on order from a female cousin of Father's. Father inherited the chairs, and he passed them on to Joe, who passed them on to me. The female cousin was the last survivor of the branch of the family to which the famous Dr. Webster belonged.

Dr. Webster became famous when he murdered Professor Parkman of Harvard University, to whom he owed large sums of money. He cut the professor into small pieces and shoved him into the furnace of the chemistry laboratory

93

at Harvard. Nothing remained of Professor Parkman but his gutta-percha false teeth. The ensuing trial revolved around an interesting point: Did the false teeth constitute a corpus delicti? The Court decided that they did, and Dr. Webster was duly hanged. To live down the disgrace, his branch of the family moved to the Canary Islands. It is not everybody, I think, whose dining room chairs have such an interesting provenance.

Curiously enough, objects like the dining room chairs or the export china took on a new meaning for me after I was told that I had an inoperable cancer. I suppose I took a new interest in my ancestors when I learned that I was statistically likely soon to become an ancestor myself.

Much the same thing happened to Father when he became an old man. After he was seventy, he spent a good deal of time trying to find out more about his forebears. He wrote to two genealogical experts in England, and they agreed that the Alsops came from a small village called Alsop in Derbyshire. But they agreed on nothing else. One wrote that the original Alsop was one Alsop-le-dale, a knight who accompanied William the Conqueror to England. This was the version Father preferred. The other genealogist wrote that the name Alsop was apparently derived from Ale-shop and that the closest thing to a family motto he could find was: "The Alsops rode to wealth on a beer-barrel."

Although I like the things in the Washington house, the house itself is a bore, like Churchill's pudding. The house I love—Tish loves it too—is Needwood Forest, Needwood for short. As soon as John Glick sprung me from NIH, I wanted to get out to Needwood, to rest my soul, and Tish and I spent all the time we could there, until I got sick again in September.

Tish found Needwood Forest. For that matter, she

found Polecat Park, which made Needwood possible. In 1950 we decided we wanted a place in the country as a weekend refuge for our growing brood—Joe, Ian, and Elizabeth were all small children then, with Stewart soon to arrive.

Tish wanted a country place more than I did, which gave me bargaining power. I drew a circle on a map, thirty miles out from the District of Columbia line, and told her if she could find a house we could live in, with not less than 150 acres, I would pay a maximum of $20,000 for it.

This sounds like a joke today, of course, and even then it meant buying a run-down farm, a rural slum. Tish was indefatigable, and eventually she came upon Polecat Park, in Howard County, Maryland—160 acres at $100 an acre, with the house thrown in. The house was a frame house, with running water pumped up from a spring and a bathroom of sorts, which also served as a hallway between bedrooms. So for $16,000 we bought Polecat Park—we so christened it because we discovered, when we had the house rewired, that seven skunks had taken up residence in the basement—and for a long time we didn't regret it at all.

I was thirty-six then, and Tish was only twenty-four, and the children were very young. For a long time we all loved Polecat Park, except perhaps for Elizabeth, who one summer, just as she was about to sit down, found a black snake coiled in the toilet, for relief from the heat. She never fully recovered from the trauma.

The house was a strikingly unhandsome house—poorfarmhouse-basic—and the land was badly farmed on shares by a country slicker. The pump kept breaking down, the heating was inadequate, and the termites got so bad by the mid-fifties that I put my foot through the living room floor. And yet, for a good many years, we loved the place. I

95

loved the place especially, because I especially needed the place.

For twelve years, from 1946 to 1958, Joe and I collaborated on a four-a-week column for the now-defunct New York Herald Tribune syndicate. Writing a political column is like climbing a ladder which has no end, and you can never see more than one or two of the rungs ahead. When nothing very much is going on, writing a political column can be agonizing—you reach up for the next rung, and there isn't any. During the two Eisenhower administrations, there were many long placid stretches when hardly anything at all was going on. There was therefore hardly anything at all to write about, and thus no rungs on the ladder to grasp.

There was another reason why I especially needed the place. Brother Joe, who had written a successful column with Robert Kintner before the war, was the senior partner in our partnership. Since I'd never written a word for a newspaper, it was an act of remarkable generosity on Joe's part to offer me a partnership after the war. (Asked by ambitious young would-be journalists how to become a political columnist, I always reply, "Have a brother who already is one.") If the offer had not been made, I would have ended up as a Foreign Service Officer in the State Department—I had filled out an application. I might be Ambassador to Chad or the Central African Republic by now, or I might not. In either case, I am quite sure I would have been miserable. Instead, despite those occasional missing rungs, I have thoroughly enjoyed a quarter century as a political journalist, and I am eternally grateful to my brother Joe for giving me the opportunity to become one, more or less overnight, without the grueling apprenticeship most political journalists undergo.

Joe is a genius, in the correct meaning of that word, and like most geniuses he is not easy to work with. He seemed to feel a psychic need for at least one shouting, foot-stamping row per week. The strains and tensions of our combative partnership, together with all those missing rungs on the columnist's ladder in the placid Eisenhower years, made Polecat Park a psychic need, a necessary refuge, for me.

By the early 1960s, all that had changed. Joe and I had had an amicable divorce in 1958. I had become Washington editor of the *Saturday Evening Post*, where I made more money than in our partnership, and where there were few strains and tensions—too few for the magazine's good. Washington had become a much pleasanter place to live, at least for a political journalist. The Kennedy people were a greal deal more agreeable and conversable than the Eisenhower people, most of whom were worthy but stuffy. And in John F. Kennedy's 1,000 days there was always plenty to write about—the ladder never lacked for rungs.

So, for me, Polecat Park ceased to be a psychic necessity. For Tish, the primitive housekeeping that had been rather fun in her early twenties became a bore and a chore. For the older children, Polecat Park became less and less a fine place for messy living and muddy swimming, and more and more a tedious place where there were no contemporaries and nothing much to do.

So we used Polecat Park less and less. I felt rather guilty about it. Becoming disenchanted with a place you once hugely enjoyed is a bit like falling out of love, a process which always engenders some sense of guilt. In any case, by February 1969, when Tish saw the ad for Needwood Forest in the *Sunday Star*, we were all rather bored by Polecat Park, except for Nicky. Nicky was nine years old

97

then, just the right age for messy living and muddy swimming, and he adored the place. He still speaks of it with the aching nostalgia of the young.

The ad in the *Sunday Star* sounded too good to be true. There was a dim picture of a big handsome house. It was described as a completely modernized historic federal house with the original paneling and seven working fireplaces, thirty acres of land, and a stocked pond. It was about fifty miles out, in Frederick County, Maryland, and the price sounded surprisingly reasonable. There was something wrong somewhere, I told Tish—it was probably one of those sad old places completely engulfed by ticky-tacky developments. But it was a dreary Sunday afternoon, and we had nothing to do, so on impulse we called the real estate agent and made an appointment to meet him at a Howard Johnson's near Frederick.

We followed the agent over a low mountain range— the Catoctins, where Franklin Roosevelt built his Shangri-la, now Nixon's Camp David—and into a valley ringed by another mountain range, with a gap in the middle. The gap was the Harper's Ferry gap, where much history was made, with the Blue Ridge Mountains to the south and Green Mountain, of Civil War fame, to the north. Instead of the expected ticky-tacky developments, there was rich, rolling farm land. We approached the house between two pillars topped by mossy stone squirrels, through ten acres of woods that had never been cut over (some of the oaks were certainly there when George Washington visited Needwood). As for the house, Tish and I fell deeply in love with it— much more deeply than with poor old Polecat Park—even before we went in the front door.

The house is a long, plain, handsomely proportioned Georgian brick house, with a tower at one end, which lends oddness and originality. The tower is unpainted, but the house itself has been painted and repainted innumerable times since it was built in 1808, and the result is a kind of patchwork of light, ochre-ish brown, very much like the prevailing color in the older parts of Rome. The agent said apologetically that "you can get this old paint blown off for around a thousand." We had no intention of following this blasphemous suggestion, but to increase our bargaining power, I agreed that this added expense would no doubt be necessary.

Inside, the house was country comfortable, with a big living room with two fireplaces, a big dining room, a nice little library, and, behind, a huge country kitchen, modernized, but with the vast fireplace where meals were cooked, we learned later, right into the 1930s. Upstairs, we counted six bedrooms, including one enormous master bedroom with two fireplaces and a bath of its own. Out back, there was a lawn and an overgrown garden and a pretty ochre-colored cottage, which we were not allowed to inspect because an old man was living in it with his angry dog.

We both knew right away that we wanted the place, but before making an offer we asked my brother Joe, who knows a lot more about old houses and the like than we do, to have a look at it. Joe is very shrewd in most ways, but occasionally surprisingly undevious. We had had one previous experience of showing Joe around a place we were thinking of buying, a big Georgetown house we were considering in 1950, when our ever-expanding family was making the walls bulge at our Dumbarton Avenue house.

On that occasion he kept saying in the presence of the agent that the place was a marvelous buy and that we ought to snap it up instantly. This precluded all hope of bargaining, of course, so we asked Joe to be sure to make no enthusiastic noises about Needwood Forest within the hearing of the agent. Joe almost overdid it. He prowled about the place, making disparaging remarks about the woodwork and the overgrown garden and discerning much evidence of termites. But as soon as the agent was out of earshot, he grabbed me by the arm and said, "Buy it, Stew, and don't haggle. It will make Kay and Polly jealous."

Katharine Graham, publisher of the *Washington Post* and *Newsweek,* has a very large and comfortable place in Virginia, and Polly Wisner, a leading Washington hostess and an old and dear friend, has a handsome farm on the Eastern Shore. The prospect of making them both jealous was vastly pleasing. Alas, they have never shown any evidence of jealousy, although, at least architecturally, Joe was right—they ought to be jealous. I did haggle the price down a bit, and because of the real estate boom in Howard County, dear old Polecat Park turned out to be almost as good an investment as Polaroid or Xerox, so that there was enough left over for a tennis court and a plastic swimming pool.

The house, it turned out, had been built by Thomas Sim Lee, second governor of Maryland and a relation of the Virginia Lees. The house had been occupied by successive generations of Lees until 1950, when Miss Gertrude Lee (who as this is written is very much alive) sold it to Colonel and Mrs. James McHugh. I have sometimes wondered if the ghostly generations of Lees resented the McHughs and ourselves as interlopers. The Lees, to judge by their headstones in a nearby graveyard, all lived to extreme old age. Colonel McHugh died of a heart attack in his fifties, and Maxine McHugh, a charming woman who made a lot of money in the forties and fifties writing best sellers with titles like *Sex and the Adolescent,* got encephalitis and had to sell the place.

After we bought it, Tish's arthritis in her hip got so bad that she was almost crippled, and it was increasingly clear that she would have to have an operation. (The operation, in the autumn of 1971, was a success.) As for myself, after that day in July when John Glick quoted the odds to me, I knew in my mind that I would almost certainly die quite soon, but in my heart I refused to believe it.

FELIX FRANKFURTER once said of a man he did not admire, "His weakness is"—here Frankfurter paused, searching for the *mot juste*—"weakness."

Weakness was also my weakness when I was discharged from NIH on a wait-and-see basis. My blood counts were low, very low, in all three vital categories, and all through August they sank gently lower. I was, in short, very sick, dangerously sick, although if I had caught a galloping infection or if I had begun to hemorrhage—the chief dangers —John Glick would have whisked me into NIH for a course of cidal antibiotics or for transfusions.

Oddly enough, throughout this period when I was very sick, I didn't feel very sick. When I came home, Andrew announced to Nicky that "Daddy is a little bit sick." A little bit sick was just about the way I felt. Sick enough not to want to play tennis (though I tried rallying a little with Tom Braden one weekend) and to want to sleep a lot, especially in the afternoon, and not to want to eat much (I began to lose a lot of unneeded weight). Sick enough not to work as hard as I ought to have worked, and to get to the office late or sometimes not at all. But by no means sick enough to give up and get into bed and wait to die.

102

It was a queer month, that month of August, a half-forgotten month, a half-alive month. I wrote a couple of columns for *Newsweek*, and we spent a pleasant weekend at Polly Wisner's place on the Eastern Shore—lots of bridge, no tennis for me—and several long weekends at Needwood. Outwardly, Tish and I and the children lived just about as we had lived before my sentence was pronounced. But there were inward differences.

For one thing there was the temptation to let things slide, to say "the hell with it," to succumb to what the French call *"je m'en fichisme."* After all, why make an effort, especially since, with a low hemoglobin count, an effort is that much harder to make?

In this respect, my friend and fellow columnist Rowland Evans was a great help. A columnist must be a reporter first, last, and all the time. Walter Lippmann wrote the best straight think-pieces, or thumb-suckers as they are called in the trade, of any journalist of our time. But even Walter Lippmann was a reporter as much as a thinker. As he wrote in his *envoi* to Washington:

> More and more I have come to wish to get rid of the necessity of knowing, day in and day out, what the blood pressure is at the White House and who said what and who saw whom and who is listened to and who is not listened to. The work of a Washington columnist requires that kind of constant and immediate knowledge. . . .

In fact, Walter Lippmann was able, for long stretches of time, to write perceptive and interesting columns from his place in Maine, far from the madding world. But when he was in Washington he made a very great effort to achieve "that kind of constant and immediate knowledge." For lesser journalists like myself, to see and talk with people, especially

103

knowledgeable people, is far more of a necessity than for a Walter Lippmann. All too often, when I try to do a thumb-sucker, I find my thumb empty of anything worth sucking. As my spirits and my hemoglobin sank, throughout that month of August, I was constantly tempted to forget about reporting, to stay home and mope. That was where Rowland Evans was such a help.

He would call once or twice a week, tell me it was time to get off my ass, and summon me to reportorial lunches, a Washington journalistic institution. The lunches, my calendar shows, were with people like Arthur Schlesinger and State Department intelligence chief Ray Cline; or with Edmund Muskie's political manager, Jack English; or with Scoop Jackson's adviser, Hy Raskin; or with Kissinger aide Winston Lord; or with various useful diplomats; or with other "sources," as they're known in the trade.

In this way Rowly Evans helped to keep me journalistically alive, and I am duly grateful. Among his fellow journalists, Evans has a well-earned reputation for competitiveness. This has never bothered me, since I am not uncompetitive myself, and on several trips we've taken together—to Eastern Europe, to Russia, to Vietnam—he's always been an entertaining and agreeable companion. But that August I was surprised to discover how *nice* he is. There is no other word for it. It sounds a bit fatuous to say so, but one compensation for getting really sick is the repeated discovery that people are nicer than they seem to be.

People are also curious about those known to be in danger of dying. Perhaps it is some sort of transferral syndrome—"there but for the grace of God go I." I looked healthy. My face is naturally pinkish, low hemoglobin or not, and I'd lost a lot of unnecessary weight. Friends and acquaintances would come up to me in a restaurant or in the Metropolitan Club, where Evans and I ate most of our reportorial lunches, and peer at me with covert intentness. Then they would tell me how well I looked, in a tone of mixed congratulation and surprise.

Obviously they had expected more outward and visible signs of moribundity. But although I looked well enough to surprise friends and acquaintances, I felt just barely "so's to be about," in the New England phrase of my youth. And as I waited for "the nature of the disease to declare itself," in John Glick's phrase, there was another inward difference. For there was always a little pea of fear at the back of my mind. It was the fear of death.

Most people have experienced the fear of death at one time or another—in combat, or at the moment of collision on a highway, or in the air, when something has gone seriously wrong. That kind of fear is sudden and sharp, with familiar symptoms—the quickened pulse rate, the sweating of the palms. This was different. It was always present, like a kind of background music. Sometimes it receded almost into inaudibility, and then sometimes it would come blaring back, accompanied by a sense of incredulity. "My God, I really *do* have cancer, and I really am going to die."

The fear leaps out, every fourth page or so, from my notebooks. An old notebook is like an old diary. Sometimes it is surprising, sometimes it is incomprehensible, sometime it is embarrassing, and sometimes in a few words it brings back vividly what had been wholly forgotten. For example:

"Nixon as peace President . . . an Ike type could have won hands down. . . . Basic weakness . . . Ike . . . cookout . . . the sleepers all favor Nixon."

Obviously I was ruminating about a *Newsweek* column that never got itself written. The phrase "Ike . . . cookout" was meant to recall an experience I had when I first began polling with Louis Harris back in the 1950s.

105

Walter Ridder of the Ridder papers and I had tried our hands at a little do-it-yourself poll-taking in the fall of 1952. We had wandered over the back country of Minnesota and Iowa in a hired car, stopping at farms to ask questions about the election and to "test farm sentiment." We both got about the same result: Eisenhower, 6 percent; Stevenson, 3 percent; Don't know, 20 percent; Ain't a-gonna tell ya, 31 percent; None of your damn business, 40 percent.

I recounted this sad tale to Louis Harris, and he offered to show me the professional technique. The technique involved adopting the costume and manner of some minor bureaucrat, say a sewer inspector, and asking all the easiest questions first, in a no-nonsense, professional tone of voice. Walter Ridder and I had tried to be too pally.

In 1956, after I had learned the sewer-inspector technique, I was polling in the suburbs of Chicago when I came on a jolly-looking fellow raking leaves in his back yard. I went through the usual easy, softening-up questions, as I had been taught by Lou Harris, and came to the crucial question: Would he vote for Eisenhower or Stevenson?

"Oh, I'll go for Ike," he said. "I know he's been sick, and he goofs off a lot—sometimes seems like he's hardly minding the store. But he's the kind of guy I'd like to invite over for a cookout. Can you imagine inviting that Adlai for a cookout?"

Ever since I've applied the cookout test to Presidential aspirants. Nothing is more obvious than that Richard Nixon fails it even more abysmally than Adlai Stevenson did. His inability to arouse the kind of personal affection lots of voters felt for Dwight Eisenhower or John Kennedy has been from the beginning his greatest source of political weakness. But it was true that all the sleepers—the hidden factors, like the race factor—then favored Nixon.

Lou Harris claimed that, using his polling technique, he never got a refusal, and when we went polling together, he proved his point, though sometimes he had to be quite astonishingly persistent to keep his record clean. In 1956 we went polling together in the Detroit area, soon after President Eisenhower's heart attack. On that expedition, as almost always when I went polling, I discovered something I had not known before. I had supposed, logically enough, that Ike's heart attack would reduce his vote, since a lot of people would realize that they might really be voting for Richard Nixon. I discovered instead that the heart attack was a major asset. We polled dozens of people who had been inclined to vote for Stevenson but had decided to vote for Eisenhower after the heart attack, for the same reason that people send flowers to a sick friend.

I also discovered just how persistent Lou Harris could be. We were polling toward dusk in an upper-middle-income suburb—ranch houses, neat lawns. Following a rule that Lou had laid down for esoteric professional reasons, we were ringing doorbells of every third house. We came to a house with a picture window, and through the window a couple— a burly man and a pretty girl—were eminently visible, in a passionate embrace on the sofa.

"Let's skip this one," I said.

"Certainly not," said Lou, and gave the doorbell a strong, demanding ring. Nothing happened. Lou rang again. The door opened, and the burly man appeared, hair disheveled, face pink with fury. Lou told me later that he recognized him as a famous professional football player of the era. Lou instantly started out on his no-nonsense, low-key spiel, adopting his incomparable sewer inspector's manner.

Slowly the pinkness left the football player's face, and

in time Lou had him answering every question. "Well, now, the way I see it is this . . ." Lou polled the pretty girl too, so we scored a double.

I became fascinated by polling as a reportorial tool. You find out all sorts of things, you didn't know before, including the fact that political journalists are writing for not more than 5 percent of the population. The other ninety-five percent don't give a damn about politics—at least the kind of detailed who-did-what-to-whom politics most political journalists write about. My brother Joe became fascinated by polling too, and we did a great many—too many —polling columns in the 1950s.

The late Edwin Lahey, a witty journalist, remarked that the Alsop brothers' passion for polling reminded him of the story of a racetrack tout who had never left Manhattan until he had had to travel to California and back to claim an inheritance. On his return to Mindy's, his fellow touts asked him what it was like out there.

"You ain't gonna believe this," he said, "but the whole goddam place is fulla people."

The story amused me—more, I think, than it amused Joe. But polling is serious business; it is a hard, footsore day's work to interview fifty people, if you are serious about it. As middle age and fallen arches crept ruthlessly upon us, both Joe and I became decreasingly fascinated by polling. But in 1960, two years after our amicable divorce, we decided to mount a joint polling expedition for auld lang syne. John Kennedy and Hubert Humphrey were locked in dubious battle in the key Wisconsin primary, and Joe and I went out to feel Wisconsin's pulse.

Joe is a journalist of commitment; he feels strongly about men and issues. He felt strongly about John Kennedy, whom he admired "this side of idolatry"—and not much this side. Joe is also an egregious fellow, in the true meaning of the word: *ex grege*, outside the flock. On that Wisconsin polling expedition, he displayed both characteristics.

It was bitterly cold in Wisconsin in early April—snow still lay on the ground. Joe had recently returned from Russia, where he had visited Siberia in midwinter. In preparation for the trip, he had had an enormous fur hat made for him in Paris. For the polling expedition he donned this fur hat and a vast, fur-lined coaching cloak that had belonged to our Grandfather Robinson. In this costume Joe looked like an angry, large-nosed, bespectacled animal peering out from behind a bush.

We trudged up through the snow to the door of our first house, a white clapboard lower-middle-class house on the outskirts of Wausau. Joe rang the bell and stood poised with his list of questions clamped to a clipboard. The door opened. An Irish-looking lady took one long, amazed look at Joe.

"Holy Mary Mother of God!" she cried, and slammed the door shut.

Joe turned to me, equally amazed.

"What in heaven's name ails the woman, Stew?" he asked, in honest bewilderment. Joe is often oddly unaware of his own oddity.

Faithful to Lou Harris's rule, we trudged on to a similar house, three doors away. Again Joe rang the bell. A lady who, to judge from her accent, had arrived on these shores less than a year before, answered all Joe's questions faithfully. She seemed quite unfazed by his peculiar costume; perhaps in whatever part of Eastern Europe she came from, the men sensibly wore a lot of fur on cold days. Joe asked his questions in an accent which, like just about everything about him, is *sui generis*. It is not quite Harvard-New England, and it is not quite Oxford-English, but it has overtones of both.

As he finished the interview, Joe clamped his clipboard with satisfaction and smiled warmly at the Eastern European lady—she was strongly for Kennedy. This emboldened her to ask a question which had no doubt been preying on her mind throughout the interview.

"Ascuse me, meester," she said. "Why you spik so broken?"

Joe looked at her in wild surmise, muttered something, and turned away.

"What in heaven's name could she have meant, Stew?" he asked plaintively, as we plowed on through the snow to a house three doors away.

The lady who answered the door was a native Midwesterner, to judge by her no-nonsense, somewhat adenoidal accent. She answered all the softening-up questions briefly; she had, it turned out, voted Democratic regularly. Then Joe came to the key question:

"In this primary election, madam, do you intend to vote for Hubert Humphrey or John F. Kennedy?"

"Well," she said, "I don't go too much for that Humphrey—he talks too much. But I guess we'll vote for him. We're Lutheran, you know, and we could never vote for a Catholic."

Joe coldly but courteously completed the interview, and we turned to go.

"Thank you, madam," he said. "I think you're a GODDAM BIGOT."

As I say, Joe is an egregious fellow, and a journalist of commitment. There are people and places who defy description. London's now-defunct Cavendish Hotel was one such place, for example. No one has ever quite caught the

110

peculiar, otherworldly quality of Rosa Lewis's Cavendish, though Evelyn Waugh came close in his *Vile Bodies*. Joe also defies description, although a good many writers have tried. But the story of our polling expedition may suggest why Joe is such good company, and why to a great many people there is an oddly endearing quality about him.

To return, after a long digression, to the August notebook, with its peculiar mixture of notes about me and leukemia and notes about the country and the world—some of the notes are incomprehensible. There are, for example, scribbles about wigs which I can't decipher; I recall only that I had decided, if I had to go into chemotherapy and lost my hair, to wear a candid wig, possibly green or pink. There are scribbles about SS-9s, SS-11s, and other Soviet missiles. Among the missiles scribbles, there is an ink outline of Andrew's hand. He likes to have his hand outlined, and his hand was small enough to get all but the tip of the thumb on a page of my notebook.

On the facing page there is an attempt to spell the name of a Polish diplomat Rowly Evans had summoned me to lunch with. Then the pea of fear surfaces in a scribbled quotation: "Dreadful is the mysterious power of fate. There is no deliverance from it by wealth or by war, by walled city, or by dark, sea-beaten ships."

Immediately below is another scribble: "38 percent abnormal cells, unidentified." This recorded the result of a marrow test John Glick gave me in the NIH leukemia clinic on August 12. I went to the leukemia clinic every few days for finger sticks or, more rarely, marrow tests. I became very used to the clinic, and I grew to hate the place.

The leukemics come into the clinic on a regular schedule for blood tests, marrow tests, booster shots of drugs, and consultation with their doctors. There is a waiting space in the clinic, with rows of chairs with plastic seats and coffee and cookies courtesy of the U.S. government. The leukemics sit there, patiently reading or chatting a little, waiting to be summoned for chemotherapy or to be told the results of their blood or marrow tests. I called the people in the waiting space the Nos Morituri Brigade. The adults, with acute myeloblastic leukemia, were all virtually certain to die of leukemia, some very soon.

Most of the children had acute lymphoblastic leukemia (ALL). There was something very hard to take about the small rows of childish faces, often topped with wigs, and the wailing that was almost always going on, of children being given marrow or blood tests. And yet this is a genuine area of hope. ALL remains the greatest child-killer of all diseases, but even since I got sick, the survival rate has improved dramatically. About half the children with ALL now live for five years or more, and a high percentage of these are considered cured—their average life expectancy is as high as that of a normal child their age.

The August 12 marrow test was a nasty one. To get spicules, John had to go into the bone twice, the second time with the largest of the marrow needles. He showed it to me afterward; it was more a tube than a needle. Mrs. Crum helped, though. Mrs. Crum is a veteran nurse, and a nice woman. I had gotten to know her in 13E, where she had told me about her favorite saint, Saint Polycarp. Mrs. Crum's theory is that Polycarp is so obscure a saint that he needs all the business he can get, and therefore he gives better service than the well-known saints. While John went into the bone the second time, she held my hand and we talked about Saint Polycarp. On the second try the technician announced that he had enough spicules for a good reading.

I am not a reporter for nothing, and by this time I knew that John expected a "fulmination" of the abnormal cells, at which point the disease would "declare itself" as undoubted AML. I waited in the usual agony of suspense for a couple of hours, and then John telephoned with his rough estimate of the results. He reported that the slides were essentially unchanged. The final count—38 percent abnormal—came a few days later. At least, no fulmination.

On August 31, in the morning, Tish drove me to NIH for another marrow test. I suddenly thought I knew what the results would be. I can remember precisely when I had this knowledge. On a corner about a hundred yards from the entrance to the leukemic clinic, there is a well-tended little triangle of roses.

"Pretty," I said.

"Yes," Tish said.

"I wonder why they don't have Japanese beetles," I said. Japanese beetles, from midsummer on, destroy every rose at Needwood. They are the bane of my limited horticultural existence. I have tried everything from the most lethal sprays to an organic grub-killer called Doom to control them. Nothing works.

"Perhaps it's because they're in the city," said Tish. "They don't seem to have Japanese beetles badly in the city."

There was a moment's silence. And then I knew that I wouldn't see the roses next year. Suspecting what John suspected, I knew—or thought I knew—that the marrow test would show a sudden sharp increase in the malignant cells. I knew that John would tell me, in his kindest way, that I would have a course of chemotherapy, and that after that I could live "a normal life." And I knew that I would have a relapse and die.

I reached out my hand for Tish's. "I have just now run

out of my small store of courage," I said. She squeezed my hand and said nothing.

A man's reaction is always mixed. I had two layers of fear. The first layer was the simple fear, that anyone who has been to the dentist knows, of being hurt—the marrow test was sure to hurt a bit, and it might hurt quite a bit. This first superficial layer of fear triggered, I think, the second layer, the underlying fear of death.

It was not, after all, an irrational fear. The blood is the mirror image of the marrow, and my blood was in very bad shape. The blood test came first. I didn't have the usual prick with the rest of the Nos Morituri Brigade; instead, John, who wanted to do some more esoteric tests, drew a plastic container of blood out of my arm. Then he "marrowed" me. The marrow test wasn't too bad, and he got spicules on the first try.

As always, the results of the blood test came first. John tried to sound cheerful about them, but I could rather easily tell that he wasn't.

The hemoglobin had sunk under 10 for the first time since I'd had a transfusion three weeks earlier, and the platelets were in the danger zone. But the worst was the WBC. The white count wasn't disastrous at 2,000. But the percentage of lifesaving granulocytes was so low that for all intents and purposes there simply weren't any. I was wholly defenseless against infection.

"Not too good, John," I said.

"Well, if you go too low on hemoglobin and platelets, we'll just transfuse you again—no problem," he said. "And we can go to the cidal antibiotics again if we have to. But I do wish those granulocytes were better."

"What does it tell about the marrow, John?" I asked.

"Let's wait and see," he said. "But if it looks bad, just

114

remind yourself we've got plenty of defenses left in our medical armory."

We went home, and I had a martini, and we had a bite of lunch. I didn't have the heart to go to the office and pretend I felt fine and talk about Ed Muskie's chances or what would happen after Nixon's Phase One. Keeping up a bold front can be exhausting.

Given the blood count, I expected a sharp rise in the malignant cells—a "fulmination," a word I'd come to dread. At about four thirty that afternoon, John telephoned. His first words were, "Now don't get excited about this; it may mean nothing. It probably means nothing." But I could tell from his eminently readable voice that *he* was excited.

"These readings vary widely, of course," he said, "but your abnormal cell count is down from 38 percent to 28 percent. As I say, this may mean nothing at all."

"But surely, John, it's not bad news."

"No, Stew, it's not bad news. There is some chance, just a very small chance, that it could be good news, though I don't know what it means."

I felt a sudden lifting of the fear that had gripped me by the triangle of roses and that had encompassed me, like some damp and awful blanket, all the hours since. No fulmination. No sentence of death. No doubt the drop in the bad cell count could "mean nothing at all." But I suddenly felt very gay.

I have a rule not to drink after lunch until seven o'clock in the evening—my father always told me that a man who didn't drink till seven couldn't become a drunkard. (I used to apply the rule to lunch too, but no longer.) It was only about 5 P.M. by this time, but I had a premature martini. It tasted marvelous, and low blood count and all I felt happy and well. Anyone who has ever jumped out of a plane with a laundry bag in the shape of a parachute on his back, and felt the chute open, and felt his feet hit the ground, and felt no bones broken and all well, will know how I felt after I had that premature martini.

A couple of days later, after the centrifuges and the computers had done their mysterious work, John called again. His own preliminary eye estimate had been right on the nose—28 percent abnormal cells. By this time, I noticed, John always used the word "abnormal." He used to call the cells "weirdos" or "bad ones," or sometimes "malignant cells," and I took this for a good sign. But then he added a comment that was clearly a bad sign.

"There has been a marked drop, and as I told you, that can't be bad news, and it could be good news," he said. "But I ought to tell you something else. The cells do look a lot more like classical AML cells."

The background music, the music of fear, blared high again for a moment. But I put John's remark out of my mind —an essential art for one in fear of death—and the background music became almost inaudible again.

AFTER THAT RATHER blank month of August, we had a Labor Day weekend house party at Needwood. The house was very full, so full that brother Joe slept on a mattress on the floor of the library. Kay and Rowly Evans and Kay Graham spent Saturday night, and we played aggressive bridge. (No one plays more aggressive bridge than Evans; he ululates in triumph when he makes a finesse or an opponent goes down.) The Tommy Thompsons came for Labor Day lunch—Tommy seemed much better—and so did John Glick and his sensible and entertaining wife Jane. It was a pleasant weekend, with people coming and going, tennis, drinks, laughs—the classic Labor Day country house party.

I had not been feeling especially chipper—hardly surprising, given my low blood count. I had no desire to play tennis, and I felt tired after even a short walk. But I love a country weekend, and I enjoyed myself thoroughly until the late afternoon of Monday, September 6—Labor Day.

After lunch I played a couple of rubbers of bridge, and then John Glick (who plays a fine game and likes to win almost as much as Evans) took my place. I felt queer —not sick, exactly, but queer—and I went up to our bedroom

117

and took my temperature. It was nothing much, just a bit above normal. But that small fever signaled a new and peculiar and still unexplained experience.

I mentioned the temperature to John Glick before he and Jane left, and he told me to take it again in the morning and, if it was above normal, to call him. I had a luncheon date the next day with Clark Clifford; I was writing a Vietnam piece, and I wanted to be sure I had his views straight. But driving into Washington that morning, I again felt queer—queer enough to call off the date. After telephoning Clifford, I took my temperature, found it again a bit above normal, and called John.

John told me to get into bed and stay there until that afternoon, when I was to get a count at the clinic. Tish drove me to NIH at about three. An hour or so later John called with the counts. They were all low, with the platelets a lousy 15,000. The temperature persisted, with a reading of 38.8 degrees Centigrade, meaning 101.9 degrees Fahrenheit. (NIH readings are always Centigrade.) John told me to stay in bed at home; I'd be in less danger of infection there than in the hospital.

At this point my faithful notebook fails me. There is a note about John Glick's whereabouts: "Sat. 8–11, Bethesda —call if Temp over 39.2." Opposite, there is a page with YES and NO in capitals repeated three times—I was trying to get Andrew to learn the difference—and two attempts at a capital A, Andrew's version. And there is a very bad drawing by me of a Volkswagen—Andrew likes drawings of Volkswagens—with Mummy driving and Daddy (with a very big nose) and Andrew in the back seat. Then nothing at all until a note written much later: "Session w. Glick— Now virtually convinced AML—v. toxic treatment—hair not out."

From September 7 to September 27 I was sick, sicker than I knew. Later, John Glick and Ed Henderson, in an interview about my peculiar case with Stuart Auerbach of the *Washington Post*, said that in my defenseless state there was a one-out-of-three chance of an overwhelming infection every day, and that such an infection could have killed me within twenty-four hours. I didn't realize I was in that kind of danger. But I did know I was pretty miserable—so miserable that for the first time in many years I had no impulse at all to scribble in my notebook.

My fever undulated gently between about 100 and 102 degrees Fahrenheit. I was forbidden aspirin, which can adversely affect the platelet count; John gave me Tylenol as a substitute. The Tylenol brought the fever down a point or two, but after four hours it would go up again. Twice I woke up quivering with a chill.

The night sweats started on Wednesday, September 8. I'd had night sweats before, when I was in NIH the first time, but nothing like this. After the first couple of nights, I learned to take three towels to bed with me. I would wake up dripping wet with sweat, swab myself off, take a Tylenol pill, sleep for another four hours or so, then wake up, swab myself off again, and take another pill. Tish had moved into her dressing room, and this gave me room to move from one side of the double bed to the other. When my side was soaking, I would move to Tish's side. By the time I moved back to my own side, it would be only a bit damp.

The anorexia—lack of hunger—also started that week. I hadn't had much appetite since July, but this was different. It was all I could do to swallow one scrambled egg at breakfast and to pick at my food a bit at lunch and dinner.

To my astonishment and dismay, even my evening martini revolted me, so that I could hardly gag it down. My sister, Corinne, recovered from her breast-cancer operation, came to dinner on the fourteenth. I dressed and came downstairs and behaved like an affectionate brother until we went in to dinner. The sight of the roast lamb revolted me, almost *ad nauseam,* and I had to say a quick good night and beat a retreat to the bedroom.

Tish drove me to NIH on the tenth, the thirteenth, and the fifteenth, and John tested my blood. The hemoglobin dropped steadily—10.9 to 9.7 to 9.0 to 8.3 on the fifteenth. The white blood count hovered around 1,000, and the proportion of granulocytes went down to 12 percent, virtually no protection at all. The platelets were consistently under the danger mark of 20,000; twice they went down to 15,000.

On September 13, when I went to the clinic, John told me to stop taking allopurinol. I had been taking either Benemid or allopurinol for some ten years, for high uric acid. Before I went into the hospital I took one tablet a day, on Dr. Perry's orders. John had quadrupled the dose; this is routine for leukemics, in order to prevent kidney stones.

John explained that he and Dr. Allen Rosenthal, an internist friend, had been discussing my peculiar case, and they both recalled rare instances when allopurinol had apparently been involved in causing very low blood counts like mine. As always, there was a risk involved in taking me off allopurinol, the risk of renal failure. But John decided to take the chance.

Despite the fever, the low counts, and the night sweats, I was perfectly capable of thinking and reading, although for the first time in years I felt no impulse to put words on paper. I read a lot—Edmund Wilson's *Upstate,* Trollope's *The American Senator,* Ralph Woods's marvelous *A Treasury of the Familiar,* ideal for dipping in and out of, and many other books and magazines.

Between spurts of reading, I would doze, and read my mail, and read some more, and doze again. Except for Tish and Nicky and little Andrew, I wanted to see no one. It was not so much that I was depressed; I don't remember being particularly sad, though of course I now thought I was quite likely to die quite soon. I was just indifferent. I didn't much care about anything.

On September 15, Tish took me to NIH. I had a finger stick, and my blood was in the worst shape yet, with the hemoglobin at 8.3 and the other counts in the cellar. I had a low fever, about 101 degrees Fahrenheit. John made another decision. He told me to come back into Ward 13. He would transfuse me, put me on cidal antibiotics, and give me a marrow test. I felt so awful that, for the first time, I was eager to go back to NIH.

Then we had that conversation which caused me to scribble again in my notebook about the "v. toxic treatment." He and the other doctors had discussed at length what to do about me, he said. They were all now virtually convinced that I had AML, though it was certainly a most unusual case. If the marrow test confirmed their conviction, I would be given chemotherapy, but not the kind originally planned. It would be, he said, with his usual candor, "a very toxic treatment," which of course involved considerable risk. But it offered about a two-thirds chance of a remission, and I might be relieved to hear that this particular treatment would not cause my hair to fall out. That was some recompense, but not much.

If the treatment induced a remission, he said, I could "lead a normal life for a year, maybe more." My case was so exceptional that there were some grounds for hoping that the length of remission might also be exceptional. He was, he said, more puzzled by my case than ever, and so were the

121

other doctors. But the consensus was that I had AML. If the low blood counts reflected a sharp increase in the abnormal cells, and if the cells continued to look like AML cells, the "very toxic treatment" was the logical next step.

After the conversation, for some reason, I began to scribble in my notebook again: "Wouldn't it be better to lie to patients—they would accept lies happily." Then: "Maybe it would have been better if case had been wholly typical, and I was slapped into chemotherapy before I knew what was happening." Then: "Sometimes sympathize with J. Glick. About the most difficult case in NIH history—and he suspects, rightly, it's going to be written about."

I re-entered NIH on September 16. Tish drove me over, I signed in, we left my bag in a room in Ward 13E, and I went down to the outpatient clinic for a three-bag hemoglobin transfusion. A three-bag transfusion lasts several hours, as the anonymous donor's blood drips, drop by drop, into the patient's veins. I am very allergic. Transfusions give me hives. Antihistamines are used to control the hives, and they make me drowsy, so the hours I spend being transfused are long, sleepy, itchy hours.

I was into my second bag, and I had been dozing. I opened my eyes and saw a lady with auburn hair, in a print dress, lying on a bed catty-cornered across the room. She was attached to an I.V. through a vein in her right arm. I recognized her as Mrs. X, one of John Glick's favorite patients; he had pointed her out to me in the Nos Morituri Brigade. She had AML and she had been in remission for almost two years. According to John, she lived a "normal life," taking care of her husband and her children, visiting the beach, and going to the movies, living like any other housewife. She was his prime example of why it was worth having a course of chemotherapy.

Mrs. X looked healthy enough, and she was quite a handsome woman. She had pretty auburn hair (a wig, probably) and regular white teeth (also fake?). She was getting her booster shot of drugs, she told me; she only had to come in every other week for her tests and her regular dose of drugs. We chattered in a desultory way, with long pauses, as the chemicals dripped into her veins and the blood into mine. I told her that I almost certainly had AML too, and that I would probably have a course of chemotherapy, like her. I was naturally wondering what it would be like to be in remission. Did she worry much about a relapse?

"Oh, no," she said, and there was a tone of genuine surprise in her voice. "The kids keep me too busy. I never even think about it, except just when I have my tests." She was quite obviously telling the simple truth.

It had always rather irritated me, when John Glick told me that if I went into remission after a course of chemotherapy I could lead a "normal life." Normal-shmormal, I told him. To live from blood test to blood test, from marrow test to marrow test, always knowing that the day would come when the tests would spell "death"—what kind of normal life was that? And yet it was clearly true that Mrs. X was indeed leading a normal life. She seemed quite unbothered by the sword of Damocles she must have known was hanging over her.

Was she, I wondered, very brave? Or was she simply unimaginative, and perhaps a bit stupid? Again I was reminded of the war. The bravest men were rarely intellectuals or sensitive souls. I suppose the bravest man I knew during the war was the captain who commanded my squadron in the Special Air Services, a British behind-the-lines *coup de main* outfit to which I briefly belonged.

The captain had three Military Crosses when I knew

123

him in Africa—I think a record for the British army—and he earned a Distinguished Service Order later in France. He once told me that he never felt so alive as he felt in combat and that he never thought about the danger to his own life at all, only about killing the enemy. He was certainly brave, but he was not markedly intelligent—his conversation was about on the fifteen-year-old level—and he was wholly unimaginative.

It occurred to me that the case of Mrs. X called for a rewriting of the lines from *Julius Caesar:*

> Cowards die many times before their deaths;
> The valiant never taste of death but once.

Mightn't "intelligent people" be better than "cowards"? And mightn't "unimaginative" or even "a bit stupid" be more appropriate than "valiant"? Hardly a literary improvement, but possibly more accurate. But maybe I was just being jealous of Mrs. X, who was clearly more valiant than I.

I did know one man during the war who was brave—perhaps as brave as the Special Air Services captain—and who was by no means unimaginative. After he had transferred from the British to the American army, Ted Ellsworth waged a one-man battle against a German company in France. He was put in for the Congressional Medal of Valor —he was eventually fobbed off with the Distinguished Service Cross. He was certainly the bravest of us Americans in the British army, and he proved he had a lively imagination when he put about the canard that my mother was a mud Indian.

I met Ted Ellsworth in a shower room of a training depot of the King's Royal Rifle Corps, near Winchester, Hants., early in 1942. It had been months since the British military attaché had advised me to be sure to bring my runabout, and the Japanese had attacked Pearl Harbor in the meantime. Because of the inevitable delays, I didn't put on the uniform of the regiment until April 1942. I had crossed the Atlantic in a small British freighter, one of a dozen or more in convoy. The crossing was choppy, and there were occasional alerts, but the food was good, a whisky-and-soda cost sixpence, and a steward had awakened me with tea every morning, which seemed to me a delightful practice.

When I arrived at the red-brick Victorian barracks of the regiment in Winchester, I was ushered into the officers' mess and received politely by four or five smartly dressed officers, most of whom were younger than I (I was twenty-seven). I was welcomed to the regiment, proudly shown the regimental flags and the regimental silver, and offered a ceremonial glass of sherry. I began to think that my decision to join the KRRC had been a shrewd one. This was better than Fort Dix.

I was told that a truck had arrived to take me to the training camp. We said good-bye politely—handshakes all round—and that was the last I ever saw of that officers' mess. At the wheel of the truck was a long-jawed, handsome young man in a lance corporal's uniform.

"Hi, Yank," he said, jumping down from the truck and proffering a hand with a sweeping gesture. "Jesus, you don't know what you got yourself in for."

Odd, I thought, the accent sounds like a Midwestern American accent. No doubt from the Midlands. I shook the hand.

"Those are my bags over there," I said. I thought he looked at me strangely, but he picked up the bags and put them in the truck. I climbed into the front seat beside him.

"Christ, I sure hope you've got some cigarettes," he said.

"Certainly," I said, and offered him a cigarette from my

125

crumpled pack of Chesterfields. After that he seemed oddly uncommunicative, though I did manage to elicit the fact that his name was Tom Braden.

He stopped the truck about four miles outside of Winchester, beside a slatternly wooden barracks, and led the way inside. The place was buzzing with talk, mostly in Cockney accents, but it stopped when we came in.

"This is where you sleep, Yank," said Braden.

"But where are the beds?" I asked.

He laughed a great cackle of a laugh and pointed to a bunchy bag of straw on the floor, which I later learned was called a palliasse.

"There's your beddy-bye," he said. "Want I should come and tuck you in?" He turned and departed, in what seemed to me an inexplicable huff.

The Cockneys were nicer. They told me where to go for "cha"—tea, which was the last meal of the day and where I made my first acquaintance with pilchards, a truly horrible English variety of the sardine—and after that, since I wanted to clean up, they showed me where to go for a shower.

The showers—no hot water, of course—were in an unheated shed. There were a couple of Cockneys in the shower room, plus Braden and a short man with black hair that stood up on his head like a Japanese doll's.

"Hey, Yank," said the short man, again in that puzzling accent. "I'm Ellsworth. Ted Ellsworth, from Dubuque. This here's big Tom Braden, also Dubuque. What's your name, and where you from?"

A great light shone. That had not been a Midlands accent after all.

"My name's Stewart Alsop," I said, pronouncing the name with a long A—my father had always insisted on the long A. "I'm from Avon, Connecticut."

"Alsop, huh?" said Ellsworth, pronouncing the first syllable as in alley.

"No, no, All-sup," I said, drawing out the A.

"Al Alsop from Avon," Ellsworth said loudly and firmly, pronouncing the Alsop like the Al, and Braden laughed that great cackling laugh.

For two and a half years thereafter, while I was in the British army, I remained Al Alsop, short A. Long before those two and a half years had passed, Tom Braden and Ted Ellsworth had become, as they remain, close friends, maybe my closest friends. While we were training in England, we discovered Rosa Lewis's Cavendish Hotel in Jermyn Street and had more drunken fun there—at least until my pursuit of Tish cramped my style—than most men find in wartime. Rosa Lewis had been both cook and mistress to Edward VII when he was Prince of Wales, as well as to other leading members of the Prince's Marlborough House set, and the Cavendish had once been one of the world's great luxury hotels. It was still comfortable in a raffish way —it was furnished like a rather down-at-heel English country house—and Rosa herself, in her more lucid moments, could still be wonderfully entertaining. She always referred to me as "Peebo Gardner's bastard," for some reason, while Ellsworth was "the little black man in the box room." Ellsworth was always assigned to sleep in the box, or luggage, room.

We Americans sailed together for Africa; Ellsworth smuggled a dog aboard, and the rest of us smuggled several cases of whisky. In Africa, alas, Braden and Ellsworth joined one battalion of the regiment, and George Thomson, Harry Fowler, and I joined another. We were sent as infantry platoon commanders to Italy, and none of us enjoyed it, but we all emerged unscathed. Except for Harry Fowler, we all transferred to the American forces eventually, and we remained unscathed, though Ellsworth was captured after his one-man battle with the Germans.

Braden and Ellsworth and I did not become friends right away. I learned later that Braden had reported to Ellsworth that "this Alsop is a *real* horse's ass." It seems that my manner, no doubt affected by that polite conversation in the officers' mess, had somehow infuriated him, I suppose for the same reason that the pretensions of the "Eastern elitists" have infuriated Richard Nixon, Lyndon Johnson, Barry Goldwater, and a lot of other non-Easterners. And he had been particularly infuriated when I offered him one cigarette. There was a fierce tobacco shortage in Britain, and he and Ellsworth had been reduced to hoarding butts. How I was supposed to know this I still don't know, but Braden and Ellsworth had expected me to come to the rescue with at least a carton apiece. Anyway, the first impression I had made was not good.

Ellsworth's revenge started with that "Al Alsop," but it did not end there. I was thin in those days, and my cheekbones showed. I had spent a lot of time sunning in a suntrap I had found on the deck of the freighter on the way over, and my face, naturally rubicund, was a coppery red. The rumor quickly spread in the training battalion that I had American Indian blood.

A considerable delegation approached Ellsworth for confirmation of this interesting fact.

"I say, Ellsworth," said an eighteen-year-old Etonian, who later reported the conversation to me. "Is it true that Al Alsop is a Red Indian?"

"Yes, it's true," said Ellsworth, his manner solemn. "But I wouldn't mention it to him, because he's kinda sensitive about it. Al's mother is an Indian, full-blooded. But she's not one of those fighting Indians, like an Iroquois, say, or an Algonquin. Al's mother is a squat Indian."

"A squat Indian?" said the young Etonian, surprised.

"Yeah, a squat Indian. Sometimes we call them mud Indians. These squat Indians, they make holes in the mud, and they do nothing—nothing at all, all day, except squat in the mud. Yeah. Al's mother is a squat Indian."

Being the son of a squat Indian did nothing to improve my image with my fellow riflemen. As for Mother, although she had a good sense of humor, she was not amused when, after the war, I told her about how she became a squat, or mud, Indian.

I did not realize, until I got sick, how much the war had meant to me. I am glad that none of my boys has been in a war. And yet they may have missed something all the same.

They may have missed some fun and some friendship. Wars can be a lot of fun, if you're lucky—plus a lot of boredom and misery, of course. And the friends you make in wartime are likely to be closer friends than any you make at other times. My children may also have missed finding out more about themselves, for war is a good way to find out about yourself. They may have missed something else that is useful too.

For it may be useful to face the chance of death when you are young. It helps to prepare you to face death when you are old. No young person really believes that this time will come. But it will.

THAT EVENING, September 16, after my transfusion and my chat with brave Mrs. X, I was back in Ward 13. I had a double room all to myself—I knew enough by this time to suspect that John wanted me to be alone in order to minimize the danger of infection. John hooked me up to the old familiar I.V., with two bottles of cidal antibiotics hanging on it. He explained, with his accustomed candor, that he didn't think they would do any good. If I had had a bacterial infection, he said, I would have had a much higher temperature, so he was sure I had some sort of virus, though tests had failed to confirm this conviction.

Antibiotics were of no use against a virus, of course, he said. I had not known this. Having so rarely been sick, I had never gathered the difference between a bacterial infection and a virus. When John first told me he suspected I had some sort of viremia, I asked him what new treatment there was for a virus. "Bed rest and plenty of liquid," he said. I remarked that medicine had not made any giant strides in this field since I was a boy.

That night, after Tish left, I managed to sleep fairly well, with the help of sleeping pills. But the next day I was scared again. John had said he would do a marrow test at about twelve thirty. I still had anorexia, which extended to liquor as well as food, but Tish made me two big martinis, and I managed to gag them down before John came in, and they helped to still the panic. John gave me the test on the bed; it wasn't too bad because of the martinis. But the waiting for the verdict *was* bad, as usual. Without saying anything to Tish about it, I had been asking myself the obvious question: Was it really worth going into chemotherapy, in the laminar flow room?

I had—I still have—a horror of the laminar flow room. The statistics have proved beyond question that the incidence of infection is markedly lower there, and thus the chemically treated patient's chance of survival is improved. But I suspect I am marginally claustrophobic, which is perhaps why I dislike flying, though I do it all the time. The thought of being cooped up for weeks in a tiny room sealed off from all human contact, was—is—genuinely horrible to me. Was it really worth doing, when there was about a 30-percent chance that the chemotherapy would kill me in the laminar flow room and, if I had a remission, a 95-percent chance that a relapse would kill me in a couple of years, more likely much less?

Might it not be better to resort to the bare bodkin? Or might it not be better to let nature take its course and let the inevitable infection kill me when it came?

While I was thinking these dour thoughts, Tish and I chatted, intermittently, about things that didn't interest us, as people do in such a situation. Then John Glick came in, and I could tell right away that his news was at least not terrible news.

The blood counts, he said, were not good. The hemoglobin had responded less than he'd hoped to yesterday's

131

transfusion; it was up to 9.5. Maybe it would do better the next day; he'd give me another couple of bags that evening. The white count was "pretty lousy," a total white count of 600, with 12 percent granulocytes—hardly any protection against infection. The platelets were in the danger area at 19,000.

But—and here was the good news—there had been no fulmination of the abnormal cells. The proportion was just about what it was the last time I was marrowed, about 30 percent. So no chemotherapy and no laminar flow room, at least for the time being. Also—and this was something not to count on, just to hope for—there seemed to be "increased megakaryocyte activity" in the marrow. The megakaryocytes manufacture platelets. They'd been "substantially absent" ever since I'd come into the hospital first, in July, and now there seemed to be quite a few in the marrow slides. So this just *could* be good news.

"No news is good news," runs the old cliché. Most old clichés happen to be true, and none is truer than this one, where a leukemic is concerned. A leukemic soon learns to expect the worst, because the worst is sooner or later virtually inevitable, so when the worst does not happen, that is a cause for rejoicing.

I spent another week in the hospital. John didn't believe that the antibiotics were doing me any good, but at least they provided protection against infection. Once a course of antibiotics is started, it must be completed, so I had to stay at least until September 23.

During this second go-round at NIH, there were no martini picnics with friends—and indeed, no martinis, or hardly any. My anorexia was almost total; it was all I could do to get down one boiled egg in the morning, and liquor, to my dismay, continued to disgust me almost as much as food. Except for Tish and John Glick, people disgusted me too. When Joe and Susan Mary paid a visit—I had passed the word that I wanted to see no one else—it was a major effort to be polite, though I love them both.

It wasn't that I felt desperately ill physically, or even desperately depressed. I felt, instead, a kind of weariness, a vast indifference. In my head during this time there was a sort of continual background music—or rather, background cacophony—not exactly a headache but a kind of murmuring unpleasantness. And a very bad thing happened: I could hardly read at all. After half an hour, the page would blur, and the cacophony in my head would mount from a murmur to a shout. For want of anything better to do, I watched television. It was the first time I have ever watched television for more than a few minutes at a time and, I hope, the last.

The chief danger was, of course, a lethal infection; that was why I was alone in a double room. At one point John told me that my granulocyte count was down to 40. "One envisages them," I wrote in my notebook, "the grizzled, battle-hardened survivors of a once mighty army, now reduced to little more than a platoon, marching out once again to do battle against the foe, well knowing that their cause is hopeless."

I was pretty sure by this time that my cause was hopeless too, but it didn't bother me half as much as it had during my first stay at NIH, when I still enjoyed those picnics in the waiting room, and drinking martinis, and reading, and laughing, and seeing my friends. The second time I was in NIH, I enjoyed nothing. I didn't want to die, but I didn't want desperately *not* to die. Who would fardels bear, to grunt and sweat under a weary life, if the weary life consisted of seeing no friends, and being unable to enjoy

133

food or drink, and sweating like a pig every night, and, *faute de mieux,* watching the mixture of tedium and vulgarity that is so much of television?

Before I got sick I hardly ever thought about death, because the subject is an unpleasant one. Since John Glick quoted those odds to me, I have had to think a lot about death, and I have learned something from the thinking. I learned something especially from those twenty days of unexplained viremia, or whatever it was (John Glick still does not know for sure). What I learned is something that most healthy people do not fully understand when they think about their own death.

If you are young and in good spirits and full of health, the thought of dying is not only utterly abhorrent but inherently incredible. The inherent incredibility of death to a healthy young man acts as a protective mechanism and helps to keep a combat soldier sane.

But the fear of death in battle is quite different from the fear of death on a hospital bed. It is, for one thing, much rarer. Most people do not die a violent death, whether on the battlefield or in the streets. Most people die in bed, because they are very sick or because they are very old or both. But their sickness or their oldness also acts as a protective mechanism. Sickness and age do not make death at all incredible. They do make death less than utterly abhorrent.

In short, for people who are sick, to be a bit sicker—sick unto death itself—holds far fewer terrors than for people who feel well. Both Cy Sulzberger and Bill Attwood wrote me letters in which they referred to death as the Greek god, Thanatos. It was at this point that I began to think of death as Uncle Thanatos. When I felt sick enough, I even felt a certain affection for Thanatos, and much less fear of him than I had before.

I was never "half in love with easeful Death," and I suspect John Keats wasn't either. Only a psychotic really wants to die. But at least the thought of death was more easeful, and far less terrible, than it had been. Afterward, when I felt well again and believed I was cured, the thought again became very terrible.

Part Two

WHAT I LATER CAME TO think of as the *dies gloriae* (all those boring hours of Latin at Groton popping up again after forty years) started while I was still in the hospital with my mysterious undulating fever. At the time the days did not seem a bit glorious, only a seemingly unending stretch of tedium.

As before, the faded blond lady would make her rounds every morning pricking fingers. Then the blood sample would be analyzed, and by about lunchtime John Glick would come in with the readings. I felt a bit like a compulsive gambler waiting for news of how his nags had done at the track. For a while my nags were losing every race.

The low point came on September 19, two days after the marrow test which showed 30 percent abnormal cells. My hemoglobin count was falling fast, my granulocytes were almost nonexistent, and my platelets, at 14,000, had scored a record low. John Glick talked about giving me a platelet transfusion, but remembering that "increased megakaryocyte activity" in the marrow, he decided to hold off for a day or so.

The next day, September 20, the platelets were back up

139

to 18,000, the next day to 20,000, then 23,000, 27,000, 29,000, 34,000, 39,000, and on September 27, when John decided to send me home, 45,000. As, day after day, John Glick gave me these readings, he could hardly contain his excitement; he was at least as pleased as I was. The readings meant—they had to mean—that the marrow was again doing its job of churning out platelets.

After John sent me home, I went back once a week to the clinic, usually for the eleven o'clock finger stick. Every day at that hour, the Nos Morituri Brigade sits on the plastic chairs, two technicians come in, and the brigade takes turns having a finger pricked. I would leave after the finger stick as quickly as I could, for I had learned to hate the place, because it smelt so of death. Then John would call me in the office or at home with the counts.

My first visit to the clinic was on October 1, and that was when the *dies gloriae* really began. For the counts showed that the marrow, all on its own, was turning out more than platelets. My hemoglobin was holding steady at 11.5. Red blood cells, like all cells, die and have to be replaced. So the hemoglobin count meant—it had to mean—that my marrow was churning out red blood cells fast enough to replace the dying cells.

The platelet count was up to a handsome 54,000. And for the first time there was really good news from the white cell front. The white blood count was 3,000—around half normal—and the percentage of disease-fighting granulocytes was 16, meaning that I had almost 500, close to the safety line. That was the best white count I had had since I was first hospitalized.

All these figures are as boring as figures usually are. But they were not at all boring to me. To me, they had a lovely, a lyrical, meaning. For they meant that something strange and wonderful and inexplicable was happening to my blood. They meant that, having faced death, perhaps in a short time, I now faced life, perhaps for quite a long time. No one, I suspect, who has not experienced this sort of reprieve can wholly imagine quite what it is like. It induces, for a while at least, a special euphoria, which no chemical can emulate and in which colors are brighter, and life more interesting, and dear friends dearer than ever before. As the counts rose and I emerged from the slough of despond in which I had wallowed, I felt as though I wanted to feel life with my hands, and see it, and smell it, and taste it, and breathe it down deep inside myself.

On October 6 I went to the clinic for another blood count and got more good news. Instead of scribbling in my notebook, I put a sheet of paper in my typewriter when I got back to my office and began tapping away. Like scribbling in notebooks, this is an old journalistic habit. For many years now, when I have had an important or interesting interview, I get to a typewriter as quickly as possible. Speed is essential. I have a phonographic memory, but the record fades. I can hear the person I have been interviewing talk, in my mind's ear, but only for a couple of hours or so. The rest is silence.

Starting on October 6, I got into the habit of recounting my medical experiences on the typewriter, when they seemed interesting. I would get to the typewriter as soon as possible, before the fading of the mental phonograph. I came to think of these notes as my journal.

Sometimes, and increasingly often as time went on, instead of writing about my medical experiences, I would sit down and tap out ideas or descriptions or recollections that had little or nothing to do with John Glick, NIH, or leukemia. These essays, or maunderings, or whatever they

141

are, were written at about the time they appear in the journal, but often bit by bit, over a period of time. So they are not dated.

The journal proper is, as writing, markedly inelegant. The late Martin Sommers, a great editor and a most lovable man who used to edit my articles for the *Saturday Evening Post*, had an annoying phrase he would repeat ruthlessly: "You've got to put it through the typewriter one more time." Much of the journal needs another time through the typewriter. But aside from some judicious pruning, I have left it as I wrote it, complete with inconsistent tenses and other inelegancies. In that condition it has the merit of spontaneity. The dated entries were written on the dates given, and without any foreknowledge of what was to come, although by the winter of 1972 I obviously had some dark forebodings.

I started the journal on October 6 because I wanted to get down on paper an experience I still wish I hadn't had —the experience of looking through a microscope at the malignant cells in my own marrow.

October 6—

Blood count at NIH. The count has broken all records. Platelets 84,000, up from 14,000 five weeks ago. Hemoglobin steady at 11.9. John Glick calls up in the afternoon, genuine delight in his voice—the granulocyte count is up to 750, the highest ever, from a low of around zero less than a month ago.

After my finger stick, at my urgent request, John showed me some marrow slides, including my own, which was perhaps a mistake. He first showed me the slide of Mrs. X, the woman I'd met when I had my second blood transfusion—the cheerful woman with a wig, who had been in remission for two years. He'd asked for a normal marrow, John said, but they were hard to find at NIH and this was just as good, because a marrow in full remission was almost indistinguishable from a normal marrow—there was very little to show that a fatal relapse was statistically inevitable.

Seen through the microscope at the first level of magnification, Mrs. X's marrow looked like Swiss cheese covered with caraway seeds. But with maximum magnification, the caraway seeds took on individual characteristics. The granulocytes were instantly identifiable; they looked like fat pink curly slugs. The megakaryocytes, which make the platelets, were big angry-looking red blobs—if I'd been shown the slide and had to choose, I'd have thought they were the malignant cells.

The hemoglobin cells were neat little cells, like big BBs, dyed purplish red. Then there were the myeloblasts (which would have been found in a normal marrow also; most marrows have 1 to 2 percent myeloblasts). Rather odd-shaped largish cells with little white spots, they looked a bit like salami slices. Then Glick showed me the slide of a girl in relapse—sure soon to die. There were clusters of cells, mostly myeloblasts, and big empty spaces. John didn't like the slide, said it was atypical, but there was certainly something very wrong-looking about it.

Finally there was my own last marrow, and there they were, the horrible little cells that are trying to kill me and, if one believes in the statistics, no doubt will. They were perfectly visible and easily identifiable. Some looked like salami slices that had gone partly bad—pink but with whitish-rotten tails. Others, John Glick said, looked like lymphoblastic cells; others looked like abnormal plasma cells.

"If I were Dr. Alsop," I told John, "I'd say this poor son of a bitch has three kinds of leukemia all at once." He

143

was not much amused and said that now I'd understand why my case was so hard to diagnose.

It is a strange feeling to look at the lethal cells crawling around in your own bones, big as golf balls under the microscope and, as John says, "obviously abnormal." They are obviously abnormal in the way that a plant, say, that is badly diseased is not like a healthy plant, or a piece of meat that has gone bad is not like a good piece of meat.

Why, I asked John, don't the white cells whose job it is to destroy enemy cells recognize these easily recognizable monsters and kill them? John shook his head and gave his stock reply, that whoever finds the answer to that question is a sure winner of the Nobel prize. But he added that the evidence of my blood shows that something is preventing the uncontrolled proliferation of the abnormal cells. Otherwise they would be crowding out the good cells, as in classic acute leukemia.

I half wish now that I had not persuaded John to show me my own slide. A mental image of the malignant cells haunts me, and I suspect it will haunt me for a long time to come.

Wednesday, October 13—

John Glick reported my counts today—platelets 125,000; hemoglobin 12.6; granulocytes, for the first time, over 1,000. He called the counts "magnificent," and when he used that word his voice rose in excitement almost to the breaking point.

What is happening in the marrow? The question fascinates John—and, since I have something of a stake in the answer, it fascinates me too. Originally, the next marrow test had been scheduled for Thursday, October 21, but John is so eager to find out what is happening that he has asked me to come in for a marrow test at ten thirty next Monday, the eighteenth.

John theorizes that the sudden upsurge in the good cell count in all three categories could be a strong recovery from the flu or viremia or whatever it was—a kind of counterattack. Or it could be a direct result of John's decision to withdraw the allopurinol. Or it could be a combination of the two. Or it could be something else, something we don't understand.

The great question is this: Does the sharp increase of the good cells in the blood reflect an equally sharp decrease in the bad cells in the marrow? That is what it ought to mean, but there is no way to be sure in advance, because there is no clear precedent for what has been happening to me. While there have been very rare cases where allopurinol has caused a sharp decrease in the white blood count, the decrease has not, as far as is known, ever been accompanied by what John calls "obviously abnormal" cells in the marrow.

It seems conceivable that in my peculiar case the allopurinol not only caused the sharp fall in the blood counts but also weakened Factor X. Nobody knows what Factor X really is—otherwise we would be well on the way to a cancer cure. But there must be some Factor X that resists the multiplication of abnormal cells, which are present in small quantities in every marrow.

If the upspurt of the good cells in the blood means a significant decline in the proportion of abnormal cells in the marrow, it would be possible to begin to hope seriously for a total remission. John Glick is obviously looking forward eagerly and hopefully to what he finds in the marrow. So am I. We shall know on Monday.

Thursday, October 14—

It is difficult to exaggerate the suspense as I wait for the marrow test next Monday.

John Glick used to say that my chances of escaping chemotherapy and that "necessary end" were about 2 percent. The other day, after a good blood test, he talked about a 5-percent chance. I suspect that secretly he suspects the chance may be higher.

I much admire John Glick, but I wonder if it's a good idea psychologically to cite odds to an old gambler like myself. I gave up poker after I had studied the odds—against filling a straight, for example, or making a full house out of two pairs. When I knew the odds, I became overcautious, and I began to lose. Once you know the odds, they turn against you. What you need is bull luck, plus blind faith.

If John is right about that 5-percent chance, I've bet on a 20-to-1 dog. He's rounding the turn into the last stretch, a length ahead of the favorite. But the odds haunt a man who takes odds seriously. Favorites win. Twenty-to-one dogs don't. In this kind of race, cancer is the favorite.

We'll see on Monday.

Monday, October 18—

Two p.m. John Glick gave me the long-awaited marrow test this morning. I really ought to have gone into the *Newsweek* office, to do some work on the column. But I am in no mood to work. My mind is not on the column—it is on the glass slides with bits of my marrow daubed on them that John is no doubt peering at through his microscope as I write this.

This is the big test, like final exams in school. If the test shows a marked drop in the percentage of abnormal cells, there really is hope for a cure—a word John used for the first time this morning. He is obviously hopeful, more hopeful than he likes to admit. At one point we were talking about Henderson's and his original decision not to put me into chemotherapy right away, back in June. He again called the decision "one of the most difficult medical decisions we ever made, and maybe will ever have to make." Then he added, "Of course we all thought you had AML then." The clear implication: He doesn't think I have it now.

After the marrow test, he said, "That didn't hurt much, did it?" And I agreed that it didn't. Then he told me he had used a small needle, much smaller than the needle he used before, which was almost as big as the kind of straw you use to suck up a soft drink. He explained that the big needle had been necessary because I was hypocellular—it was necessary to get a lot of the stuff to get a good sample. And even then, there was too often the dreary exchange between John and the technicians. "You have spicules?" "No, sorry, no spicules." Then John would have to shove the needle in again, forcing it hard through the backbone to get spicules—a representative portion of marrow. This time the small needle went through the bone easily, and there were spicules on the first pull.

Four p.m. John calls. I can tell by his tone that he is delighted. But he starts with bad news. The white cell count is a bit off, but this could be just a dip. The platelet count, at 180,000, is essentially normal. The red cell count is up to 12.6, also close to normal.

"Fine," I say, my voice quivering with suspense, "but what about the percentage of malignant cells?"

John has obviously been saving the best for the last, like dessert for a child: "Under ten percent." This down from 44 percent at the start.

147

Surely this could only be good news?

"Marvelous," says John. "Almost miraculous." He had told Dr. Henderson that afternoon, and the usually dour Dr. Henderson's only comment was "Wow!"

So what does it mean? What happened?

"We don't really know, of course, and we may never know. All we know is that something has happened to make you suddenly much better. It is as though there has been a big foot holding down your marrow, and now the foot has been removed."

The marrow, as John had suspected, is neither hypocellular nor hypercellular; it has a normal cell disposition. "How about those remaining cancer cells, though?" I asked. "We've still got to worry about them, don't we?"

"Well, yes," John said, "but don't call them cancer cells—they may not be. All we really know is that they're abnormal cells."

"So what does it mean? Does it mean there is a serious chance of a genuine cure?"

"An exc—"

"You were going to say 'excellent,' John, weren't you?"

"Let's say a good chance, a serious chance. You know, this is the kind of thing—well, if you have a good bottle of champagne in your cellar, this is the night to get it out and drink it."

I can't believe John would have mentioned that bottle of champagne unless he is convinced that the chance of a cure is in fact "excellent." All this, mind you, from the doctor who told me in July that I had a 50 percent chance of living a year, that it was 20 to 1 I wouldn't last two years, and that the chance of a cure was "statistically negligible."

I am not a religious man, but I think when nobody's looking I'll drop into a church tomorrow and say a prayer.

A couple of days after this entry, walking back to the *Newsweek* office from a reportorial lunch at the Federal City Club, I came to the handsome old yellow stucco Episcopal church on Lafayette Square, "the Church of the Presidents." A door was open, and on impulse I went in and sat in a pew. There was only one other person in the church, an elderly man on the other side of the aisle, on his knees, praying.

With a certain sense of embarrassment, I put my head down between my hands, as I used to do in chapel at Groton, and said the Lord's Prayer. I said it very rapidly, as I used to in the days when God was a big bearded reality to me. I got as far as "and give us this day our daily bread, and forgive us our trespasses, as we forgive those who trespass against us." Then I stopped. I couldn't remember the final words. All the time that faint sense of embarrassment persisted, the feeling I get (and so I suppose does everyone else) when I am doing something that is not quite natural.

I wish I could say that this strange experience with leukemia has given me profound spiritual insights. But it hasn't. The big bearded reality of my childhood is no longer a reality to me, which was why I felt a faint sense of embarrassment. I have been an agnostic since I was about eighteen. I am an agnostic still.

Sitting in church I remembered a few lines from a horrid little poem we used to recite as children—as with the Lord's Prayer, I couldn't remember all of it:

> The worms crawl in and the worms crawl out.
> They crawl all over your face and snout.
> They make a helluva mess of you . . .

149

That seemed to me a more likely prospect than life after death. I remembered also the words of the treacherous King in *Hamlet:* "My words fly up, my thoughts remain below."

And yet—and yet. There is that other cliché quote from *Hamlet:* "There are more things in heaven and earth, Horatio, than are dreamt of in your philosophy." I am an agnostic, not an atheist. I do not say there is no God, I say only I do not know whether there is a God. There is certainly a mystery out there somewhere.

In a way we are all religious whether we like it or not. That peculiar little incantation to God, Mother, Father, and Aggie is, I suppose, a manifestation of some sort of religion.

I have developed another incantation. It comes from an anthology of Winston Churchill's writings about America, edited by Kay Halle. Kay sent it to me when I first got sick. In one piece, written in 1932 when he was doing a lecture tour of the United States, Churchill describes how he was run over by a taxi in New York.

He had been looking for Bernard Baruch's house one evening and had got hopelessly lost—one suspects that he had drink taken. Thinking he recognized Baruch's house, he started to cross a street toward it when he was hit by the taxi and very nearly killed. He describes this experience in a plain unadorned style, and then suddenly there is this vintage Churchillism: "For the rest, live dangerously; take life as it comes; dread naught; all will be well."

I find myself repeating this Churchillian sentiment like a talisman—or, I suppose, like a prayer.

One discovers things about oneself by writing a book mostly about oneself. I have been genuinely surprised to find out how much I was affected by the war and by Churchill.

Churchill is very old-fashioned now, only a few years after his death, and the revisionists are already gnawing at his bones. Admiring him marks a man as a fuddy-duddy, the way admiring such unfashionable figures as Kipling or Theodore Roosevelt marked a man as a fuddy-duddy when I was growing up in the thirties. Moreover, I don't pretend to have read all of Churchill or even most of Churchill. Great swatches of his prose are soporific, and a lot of his rhetoric reads as though he had been immersed all too thoroughly in Macaulay and *The Decline and Fall.*

Nor is it enough that Winston Churchill was a brave man and a patriot; there are many such. I believe now, as I believed when I considered myself a "Marxist liberal," that it is far more important to have enough to eat than to have a flag to wave. In a way, I suppose, my admiration for Churchill is a conditioned reflex—Dr. Peabody and the Groton Fife and Drum Corps and some books I read when I was young, and some songs and movies and hymns, and the war and some people I knew in the war. But there is more than that—there was in Churchill's life a kind of elegant integrity. In any case my fuddy-duddy admiration for Churchill has become a part of me.

ıı

Wednesday, October 27—

Went to NIH for a blood test today. John took some blood and told me the final official estimate of the proportion of abnormal cells in the October 18 marrow test: 6 percent. Just about what he had thought—"substantially under ten percent," he had told me.

151

Dr. Allen Rosenthal, the internist with whom John first discussed the withdrawal of allopurinol, came into the clinic. We went into one of the treatment rooms and had a long talk, John leaning against the high operating table, Rosenthal and I sitting on metal chairs.

Glick and Rosenthal together seem to be more conservative about a cure in my case than Glick alone has been. John used to talk about a cure and dismissal from NIH by Christmas or even by Thanksgiving, but today they agreed that there would be no final decision until February or even March. I suspect that this relative conservatism reflects no change in my condition—it is a reflection of Allen Rosenthal's influence on John.

John is one of nature's optimists—to him, the glass is always half full, never half empty. Rosenthal is a cooler type. He is calm in manner and physically stocky, a contrast to John's intensity and wiry thinness. He has a broad, humorous face and reddish hair. I first met him in 13E when I had the flu (if that is what it was). He asked about my symptoms. I told him about the undulating fever and the night sweats and said that I also had anorexia, adding by way of explanation that "I seem to have no appetite." "Got it the first time," said Rosenthal with a grin, putting Dr. Alsop in his place.

John and Rosenthal plan a joint "case report" on Alsop's disease for some medical journal. They'll wait three or four months, until—or so one hopes and prays—two or three marrows have been normal. It is always possible, John says with uncharacteristic pessimism, that things could begin moving back in the other direction—that "one fine day we'll get a reading of 30-percent abnormal cells." But John clearly does not believe that this eventuality (which would lead me again to think long and hard about the bare bodkin) is at all likely.

John lists again "the variables"—Atromid, for high cholesterol, allopurinol, the virus attack. (John still feels sure it was a virus, though all the viral tests have come back negative.) There have been cases—very rare—of a virus causing, or seeming to cause, a spontaneous remission. But the odds against a spontaneous remission are vast.

"A thousand to one?" I ask.

"More than that," Glick says.

That leaves allopurinol as the major suspect. Allopurinol has caused pancytopenia, as well as skin rashes, unexplained fevers, and other disorders. But John returns to the basic point, as a dog to a bone. Allopurinol has *never* been known to cause obviously abnormal cells, looking every bit as malignant as proven AML cells.

The case study may thus have to record that the Alsop case is simply bizarre, wholly idiosyncratic, without any identifiable etiology. But if allopurinol can be identified as the criminal, a relapse would be very unlikely. It would be somewhat more likely in case of a spontaneous remission, since the original conditions which brought on the malignancy would continue to exist.

"Of course, if you were a dog or monkey, we would feed you progressively bigger doses of allopurinol and find out for sure in that way. But we can't do that with a human being."

Suppose it is definitely proven that allopurinol caused the problem. Will it be taken off the market?

Almost certainly not. Allopurinol, Glick and Rosenthal explain, is a very valuable drug, which has saved many lives. Chloromycetin, for example, is a valuable drug too, but because it has caused aplastic anemia in a tiny proportion of cases—one or two out of twenty to thirty thousand —doctors now prescribe it with extreme care. In the same way, if allopurinol is definitely proven to be the culprit,

153

the "case report" will doubtless lead doctors to prescribe it also carefully and reluctantly and to keep a close watch on the subsequent blood counts.

So if it turns out that allopurinol *is* the culprit, will this mean that I never really had cancer at all? Very probably. Then how to explain the seemingly malignant cells? "We would have to call them bizarre drug-affected cells, or something of the sort," John says. "Dyspoietic is the technical word. We see drug-affected cells in the marrows of patients in remission from AML. Mrs. X's marrow, for example—at first glance it looks normal, but to the expert eye there is something odd-looking about some of her cells."

The night sweats have never been explained. "I swear I didn't imagine them," I tell Glick and Rosenthal. "I'd wake up in the night half drowned in sweat."

"I know," John says. "Naturally I suspected tuberculosis—night sweats, unexplained fevers, and anorexia are all symptomatic of TB. We did every known TB test on you, and you just don't have it." There is a faint note of annoyance, as though I'd broken the rules.

Glick and Rosenthal talk about drug-induced disease. A drug called Dilantin, which is structurally related to allopurinol, has occasionally caused a condition that mimics lymphoma. The seemingly malignant lymph tumors disappear when the drug is stopped. Other drugs have caused false cancers.

"All drugs are poisons, to one degree or another," Rosenthal says. "Between twenty and thirty percent of the diseases we treat here are partly or wholly drug-induced."

"Yes, but a doctor has to be very careful talking about this sort of thing to a layman, even an intelligent layman," John says rather hastily. "Everybody has his own favorite horror story, and although it's true that pills can be poison, they have saved a lot of lives and made a lot of lives livable too. Take aspirin—a very, very useful drug. But it's also true that aspirin in some rare cases can make platelets ineffective. You'll never take an aspirin again, for the rest of your life. But because of this very rare phenomenon, are we going to outlaw aspirin? Of course not."

Rosenthal suggests that Glick look into some experiments being conducted by Sheldon Wolff of NIH, and Glick takes down the name. Wolff has been studying a canine disease called "gray collie disease." It seems that some collies are born with rather beautiful light gray coats. Kennel keepers used to kill them as soon as they were born because they always died prematurely, and the disease is genetic and thus inheritable. Then Wolff became interested in the disease and began advertising in kennel magazines. He now has a kennel of gray collies, and he has kept some alive beyond their usual short span.

Collies with "gray collie syndrome" completely lose *all* the cells in their marrow every two weeks. Then four days later the marrow mysteriously returns to normal. But of course the poor dogs are without protection against infection during the time when they have, in effect, no marrow, so they inevitably die of infection, just as untreated AML patients do. Glick is clearly much interested in gray collie syndrome—perhaps he suspects that I am some sort of gray collie in human form.

Glick, reminded by the disappearing marrows of the gray collies, begins to talk about my first marrow test at NIH. The marrows were so thin on cells of any type that they were almost like a gray collie's. The megakaryocytes, the platelet-producing cells, were "essentially absent." On the first test, they found one single megakaryocyte. "We used to joke that maybe we'd taken the very last mega-

155

karyocyte out of your marrow." (Sometimes John doesn't find my jokes very funny, and sometimes I don't find his very funny.)

|||||||||||||||||||||||||||||||||||||||||||||||||||||||||||||||||||||||||

The news that I was in NIH and that I had been diagnosed as an acute leukemic spread fast among my friends, and faster still when I wrote two pieces about the experience for *Newsweek*. I soon began to get a lot of letters.

Writing a letter to a friend who is thought to be dying is a difficult assignment, and I was interested and amused by the varying techniques several friends brought to the job. After my cousin Alice's "what a nuisance" note, perhaps my favorite letter came from Jock Whitney, whose sister Joan Payson owned the New York Mets:

> Dear Stew:
> A friend of mine was sitting next to my sister Joan at the opening of the Metropolitan Opera with Madame Callas, looking glorious, two seats away.
> The program began with the Star-Spangled Banner, at the conclusion of which Joan settled into her seat with the audible statement, "Play Ball!" Mme. Callas cracked up.
> With warmest wishes.
>
> *Jock*

A perfect letter to a very sick man, since what a very sick man needs above all is to be cheered up, and nothing is more cheering-up than a good laugh. A letter sometime

156

later from my cousin W. Sheffield Cowles, an old friend and a witty man, gave me another good laugh. Cowles had had, as he wrote, "a stroll in the valley myself"—he had had an aneurysm.

"Our Episcopal minister called on me in the hospital," Cowles wrote. "As he was leaving, he wished me luck. I said, 'Send up a prayer for me.' He came back and folded my hands across my heart, put his own hands on mine and ad libbed quite a long message to which I said Amen.

"The next day he caught up with me as I was walking down the corridor to the Can, and he asked me what church I belonged to. I said yours. He said but I've never seen you in it. I said I was in it for Dan Pierpont's funeral. He said that was twelve years ago. I said I didn't go to church often. He said but you are deeply religious. I said not really. He said you must be religious or you wouldn't have asked me to pray for you. I said to tell you the truth that was more or less like putting a chip on the double zero. After that he cast me loose to go to the Can in peace."

I had many thoughtful and moving letters from friends and from journalistic colleagues. I was touched when Teddy White—Theodore H. White of *Making of the President* fame—offered to act as my leg man for the column, if I hadn't recovered "the full vigor to tackle the road in a Presidential campaign." Journalism is a highly competitive trade, and as any journalist will agree it was a remarkably generous offer.

I was especially cheered up by a note from Ben Bradlee, executive editor of the *Washington Post*. Bradlee descends from ancient New England stock. He wrote: "I came back from vacation to hear the distressing news that you are now full of common or ordinary blood. Not that I want this bruited about, but I have a little extra, and it *is*

157

blue." This pleased me, because it gave me an opening for a crushing rejoinder: "Dear Ben. Coals to Newcastle. What cheek."

By the time I got Ben Bradlee's letter, I had begun to work on this book, and I had been wondering what to call it. Rereading my reply, a title occurred to me: "After Many a Summer Dies the Snob."

One way to cheer up a sick man is to massage his ego. I got a number of ego-massaging letters from politician friends, including one from Ed Muskie, who wrote that "I have always gained immensely from the honesty and eloquence of your writing." In the fall of 1971, Muskie seemed to have the Democratic nomination almost sewed up, and it was cheering to get an ego massage from a potential President. I got another ego-massaging letter from Hubert Humphrey, who, ideology aside, has long seemed to me about the most humanly likable politician I have known.

Another way to cheer up a man supposed to be dying is to suggest that he may fool the doctors yet and to produce substantiating evidence. John Roche, the columnist and Brandeis University professor, wrote an especially cheering letter:

> Dear Stew:
> I was terribly distressed to hear of your ailment, though glad to hear it has been tempered by ambiguity. Let me tell you a story: in 1948 my father was dragged into the hospital (he didn't believe in them, arguing that since most people died in hospitals they were places to avoid) and the wise men diagnosed terminal, inoperable cancer of just about everywhere from the belt down. They gave him up to 6 mos. and, unwisely, suggested to my mother that he not be told.

Ten years later—to make a long story short—he died of a heart attack, aged 72. When they did the post mortem, they discovered the cancer had simply died out. Of course, they went nuts trying to find out what he ate, drank, smoked, etc., etc., but to my knowledge never found much. I sometimes think he did it to fool the priest: he got the last rites about every 6 months. But like acupuncture, this suggestion was never given serious consideration by the shamen.

Admittedly my old man was a hard case, but you have always struck me as being in the same general category. So fool the bastards. . . .

Yours,

John

Jim Polling, a friend from prewar days, when we were both editors at Doubleday Doran, wrote an even more cheering-up letter. He described the case of a sixty-year-old man who was diagnosed as a leukemic and given six months to a year to live, back in 1947, and who was still breathing at eighty-three. A leukemic very much wants to hear about other leukemics who have beaten the terrible odds.

But the most cheering-up letter of all came from Dean Acheson, in response to the first column I wrote for *Newsweek,* describing the experience of being told of death's imminent inevitability.

I had been worried about the column. A political columnist is supposed to write about politics, not about himself. I was afraid above all that the column would seem sentimental, self-pitying, mawkish. And curiously enough, what made me especially nervous about the column was the thought that Dean Acheson would read it. I saw him quite often at the Metropolitan Club, where we both lunched, and he occasionally commented on a column, sometimes acidulously and sometimes with a compliment, so I knew he read what I wrote.

I admired Dean Acheson very much. I admired him when, almost alone in terrified Washington, he stood up against Joe McCarthy, and I also admired him when in his old age he stood up against the post-Vietnam neo-isolationism of many of his fellow Democrats. He was sometimes wrong, of course, like everybody else, but there was never a man who so clearly had the courage of his convictions, right or wrong. I was also a little bit scared of Dean Acheson. He detested silliness, and he was justly famous for his put-downs—when he put down a fool, the fool was left in no doubt that he was a fool.

His letter is dated 29. VIII. 71, a way of dating letters peculiar to him:

Dear Stew,
     You are one hell of a man. I am proud to know you and wish that I had half your guts. . . . May you go on to prove a miracle and live to write as wisely and sensibly as any man ever did.
     Alice sends her love.

As ever,

Dean

Dean Acheson died a few weeks later on October 12, 1971. He died the way a sensible man should wish to die. Full of years and honors, he slumped forward on his desk, without a moment's agony or suspense. Something, I think, died with him.

It is hard to define exactly what that something was,

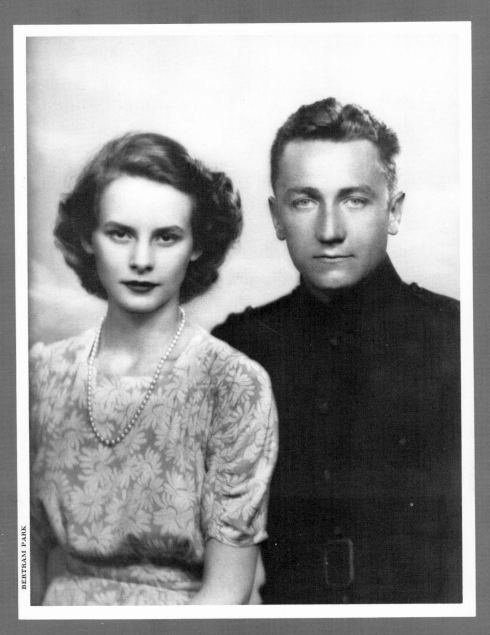

BERTRAM PARK

Miss Patricia Hankey and her fiancé,
S.J.O. Alsop, Spring 1944.

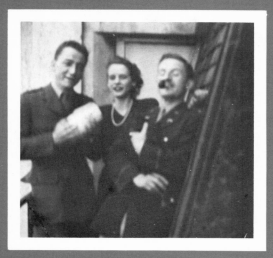

Stew, Tish, John on the roof of the Ritz — honeymoon, martinis, and buzz bomb watching. London, June 1944.

North Africa, 1943. Lts. George Thomson, Stewart Alsop, Theodore Ellsworth, Harry Fowler, Thomas W. Braden.

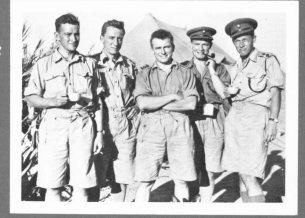

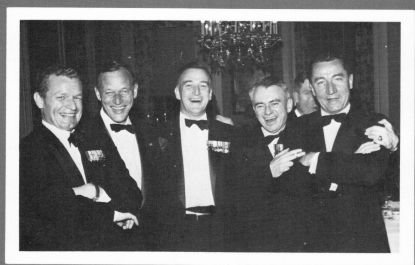

Reunion, 1960: Fowler, Braden, Thomson, Ellsworth, Alsop.

Curious Alsop custom of being photographed sideways —

Uncle Otto,
Uncle Frank,
Uncle John,
and Pa,
circa 1888.

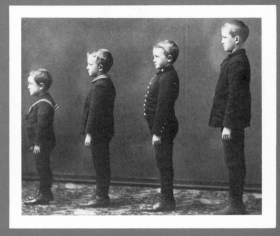

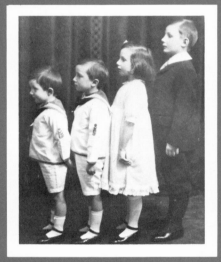

John, Stew,
Sis, and Joe,
Around 1919.

Christmas
line-up, 1956:
Stewart,
Elizabeth
(mugging),
Ian, and Joe.

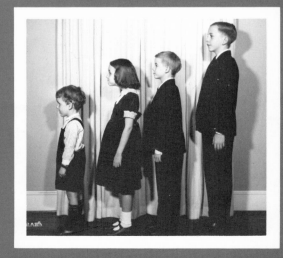

Another curious Alsop tradition.

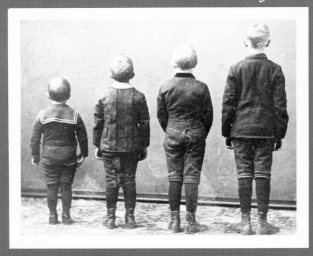

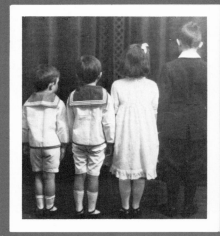

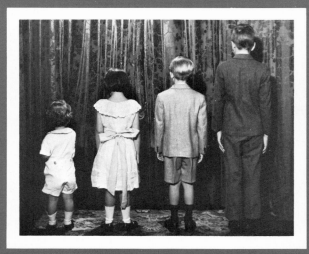

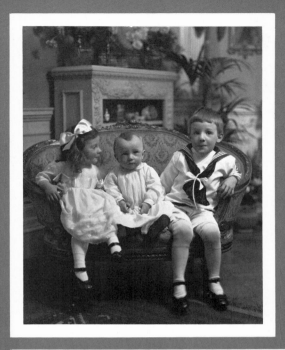

Sis, Stew,
and Joe,
circa 1915.

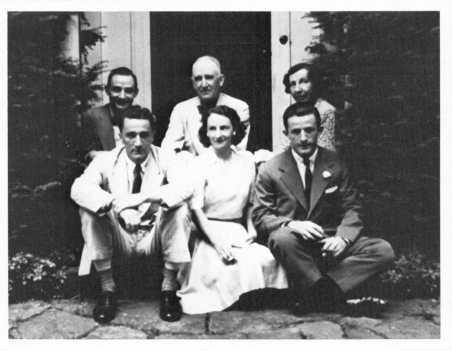

Before front door of Avon, about 1939:
J.W.A.V   J.W.A.VI   Ma
Stew   Sis   John

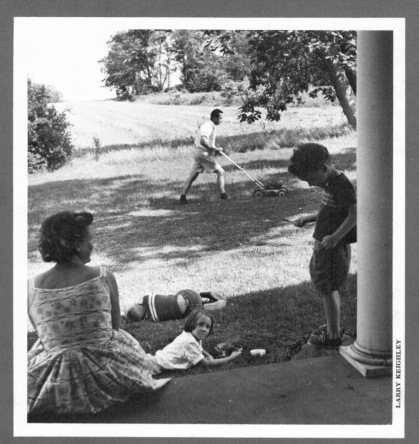

LARRY KEIGHLEY

Weekend at Polecat Park, circa 1956.

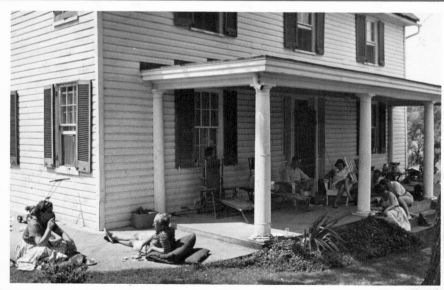

LARRY KEIGHLEY

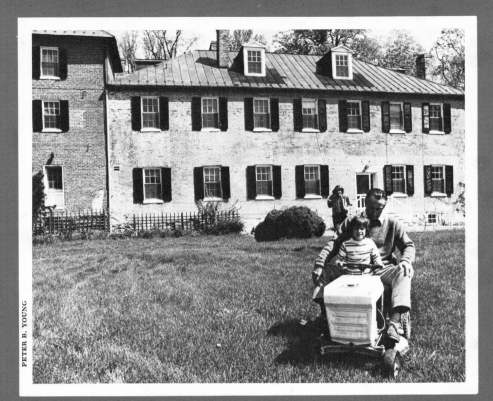

PETER B. YOUNG

Needwood, 1973. Andrew driving, Nicky behind.

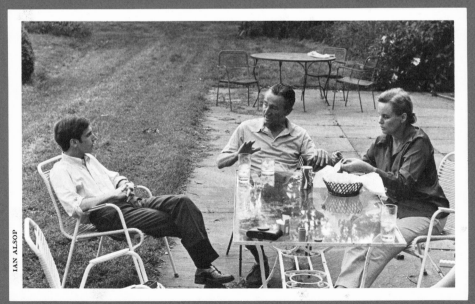

IAN ALSOP

John Glick visiting Needwood.

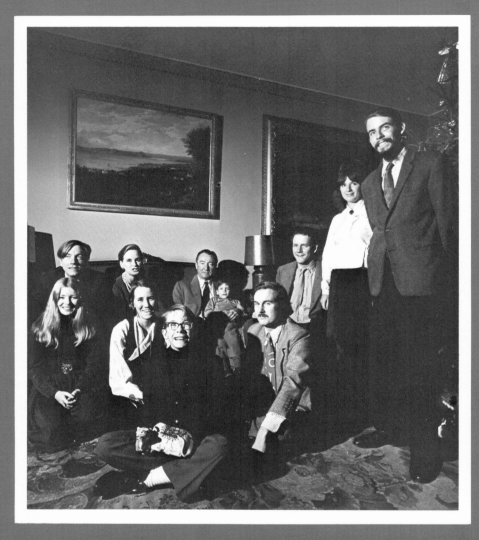

Christmas, 1971. Candy, Joe, Tish, Elizabeth, Nicky, Daddy, Andrew, Peter Mahony, Stewart, Jill Charlton, Chan.

and many people, including many highly intelligent people, are perfectly happy to see it die. I am not one of them, but then a man is a product of his conditioning, as well as his genes, and I had very much the same kind of conditioning Dean Acheson had. Acheson went to Groton and Yale, and so did I, and he was born and brought up in Middletown, Connecticut, where five generations of Alsops lived. We were both conditioned to a certain unconscious Anglophilia. So were most of the people who ran the foreign policy of the United States, from the early New Deal, and indeed from the era of Monroe and Castlereagh, until the Vietnam era.

At Groton, the sons of the Eastern Wasp establishment of Dean Acheson's day, and of my day too, were given an American imitation of an English public school education, and the same was true of the other private schools to which the sons of the establishment were sent. Something of the flavor of that kind of education is no doubt conveyed by the occasional literary references in this book—almost invariably, they are from English sources, from Shakespeare to Hilaire Belloc, from the King James Bible to that thoroughly Anglicized American, T. S. Eliot. A good many of them were learned at Groton. Most of what a man remembers he learned when young.

We worked hard at Groton, in part because there was not much else to do. And it was typical of the Groton of my day—and Dean Acheson's—that in five years there I was given five years of English history and no American history at all. It is remarkable how many men who had a profound influence on American policy were exposed to this sort of proto-English education.

Franklin Roosevelt went to Groton and so did slews of other Roosevelts, Whitneys, Morgans, and the like. Sumner

169

Welles, Roosevelt's most influential foreign policy adviser after Harry Hopkins, went to Groton, and so did Roosevelt's Attorney General, Francis Biddle. So did Averell Harriman, Douglas Dillon, McGeorge Bundy, William Bundy, most of the top command of the CIA in the Allen Dulles period, and dozens of other lesser lights in the government. In the Roosevelt, Truman, and to a lesser extent the Eisenhower period, a very large proportion of the other people who ran our foreign policy had gone to schools like Groton and to one of the three major Ivy League colleges.

All these people, I think, had been conditioned to accept two assumptions about foreign policy: (a) Great Britain was, and would forever remain, a great power and (b) when the chips were down, Britain and the United States would be allies.

People with a conditioned Anglophilia not only ran the foreign policy of the United States. In the sense that the old Wasp establishment was predominant financially and even intellectually, until recently such people largely ran the United States. They no longer do. Dean Acheson's sudden and painless death symbolized the death of the Wasp establishment, which unlike Acheson, was a long time a-dying.

The Wasp establishment began to die, I suspect, way back in the 1930s when Richard Whitney, still another old Grotonian, was photographed entering the paddy wagon on his way to Sing Sing, with his Porcellian Club pig clearly visible on his waistcoat. But the Wasp establishment first became irreversibly moribund in the autumn of 1956 at the time of the Suez crisis. The Suez fiasco was a visible symbol of the destruction of Great Britain as a great power, and the United States played a matricidal role in that act of destruction. The destruction of Great Britain as a great power in turn accelerated a process that has ended with the destruction of the Wasp establishment as the dominant source of American leadership.

When John Foster Dulles forced the British backdown at Suez, Harold Macmillan cabled his old friend Dwight Eisenhower: OVER TO YOU. His meaning was obvious: Britain was opting out of the great power role, and henceforth the United States would have to go it alone. The ending of Britain's great-power role was a tragedy for the United States, but especially for the Wasp establishment.

For it disproved a basic assumption and rendered dubious a whole way of looking at the world, and thus undermined the self-confidence of a great many people who had been taught to believe—and sometimes to believe quite rightly—that they were especially good at running the country. An elite that has lost its self-confidence soon ceases to be an elite.

Vietnam completed the process of undermining the self-confidence of the Wasp establishment. Now this country has no establishment. Perhaps it is better off without one. But I suspect not. I suspect that a great power needs an establishment, an elite, a class of self-confident and more or less disinterested people who are accustomed to running things.

At any rate Dean Acheson is dead now, and so is the Wasp establishment. American policy making is dominated, not by Waspish Ivy Leaguers like Roosevelt or Welles or Acheson or Harriman or the Bundy brothers, but by a Kissinger or a Connally or a Shultz. Maybe they will do a better job—Henry Kissinger, at least, is as brilliant a policy maker as I've seen in a quarter century of covering Washington.

Moreover, a lot of bad mistakes were made when policy

was made by the Wasp establishment, and a lot of the people who went to Eastern boarding schools and the Ivy League colleges and thought of themselves as an elite were neither as able nor as disinterested nor as elite as they liked to think. Some of them were fools.

Yet they were at least generally incapable of the kind of sleaziness, the small-minded grubbiness, that has since become so marked a feature of the Washington political scene. This is why a small tear may perhaps be shed for the death of the Wasp establishment, which breathed its last breath when Dean Acheson slumped forward on his desk.

||||||||||||||||||||||||||||||||||||||||||||||||||||||||||||||||||||||

Monday, November 8—

Last week there was a mysterious dip in the blood counts, and John told me to come in today for a blood test and then, if things look wrong, a marrow test. He drew the blood, a bit extra, since he had some esoteric tests in mind, and told me to come back in forty-five minutes, when he'd have the count and he would decide whether to go into the marrow.

I had had no breakfast, on John's instructions; the esoteric tests required an empty stomach. Tish and I wandered down to the basement cafeteria. Breakfast was no longer being served, so I had a detestable sweet roll and a cup of coffee. I was scared, for the first time in weeks, and I had trouble getting the sweet roll down. I was scared of having a marrow, and I was scared of what might follow, if the percentage of bad cells had started climbing again. Tish and I sipped our coffee and talked a bit about the news and watched the clock. At eleven, the forty-five minutes had passed, and we went upstairs to the clinic.

There was a happy grin on John's readable face. "No marrow this time," he said. The count was close to normal. "If you went to a doctor with this count, he might tell you to come back in a few weeks for a checkup, but he'd be more likely to tell you to go about your business."

I felt a flood of relief. I admitted to John that I'd been scared and asked him if he thought being scared might somehow affect the counts. He said no, but that there was no doubt that the psychological state did in some mysterious way affect the physical state.

"That's one argument, of course, for telling you nothing," he said. "That's what some doctors do, but it's not what we do here." This is a subject which clearly bothers John—he returns to it like a dog to a bone. For myself, I'm ambivalent. I like to know where I stand, but I don't at all like being scared.

Mel Elfin, chief of the Washington bureau of *Newsweek*, has warned me against *kinehora*, a Yiddish word for the kind of overweening confidence that invites the wrath of the gods. Before last's week's sinister dip in the blood counts, I was no doubt guilty of *kinehora*. I don't think I shall be again.

Two bottles of organically grown Queen Bee Jelly arrived today from England. It was sent by Rosie Baldwin, a friend from the Cavendish Hotel days. A pamphlet that came with the bottles recommends it for everything from waning sexual powers to leukemia. I have already started taking the recommended dosage, an "eggspoon full" a day.

The theory of Queen Bee Jelly interests me. It seems

173

that when a hive needs a queen, a little female bee exactly like all the other little female bees is chosen at random. She is stuffed with Royal Jelly and immediately begins to grow an enormous bottom. (I hope that doesn't happen to me.) She becomes much bigger than any other bee, lives about eight times as long, and develops prodigious sexual powers.

Rosie Baldwin writes that a member of White's Club took to eating the stuff and reported to the other members that it had endowed him with prodigious sexual powers. Now, she writes, virtually all the members are consuming Queen Bee Jelly.

Wednesday, November 17—

I had an appointment for a finger stick and a marrow test at ten thirty today. After the finger stick, John Glick led me into one of the clinic operating rooms and talked about a conference that had been held about my case. On the Friday before, it seems, there had been a national conference on acute myeloblastic leukemia, attended by some of the leading specialists in the country, including—and one sensed a certain reverence as John pronounced his name— Dr. Clarkson of the Sloan Kettering Institute.

The specialists had all had a look at my marrow slides and discussed my case. By and large, I gathered, they had been skeptical of the notion that the withdrawal of allopurinol had caused my remission. Dr. Clarkson and most of the other specialists agreed, after looking at my first marrow slides, that they would have diagnosed my case as an odd and atypical AML just as Dr. Henderson and John Glick had done. After they had looked at the most recent slides, the ones with less than 6 percent abnormal

cells and a normal cell distribution, there was much mysti-
fication, I gathered. Dr. Clarkson confessed himself as mystified as anyone else. But he hazarded a guess—that I had
had a "harbinger," or warning signal, of some sort of atypical malignancy, perhaps a "lymphoproliferative disorder,"
which I gathered was a sort of slow-growing cancer of the
lymph glands. Another specialist suggested a second look at
"some sort of atypical dysproteinemia" or an unusual lymphoma of some kind. One argument for a lymphoma, John
explained, was that the malignant cells in the marrow in
this kind of cancer can be "patchy," with big ups and
downs. Classic AML, by contrast, is never patchy; the
malignant cells have a predictable doubling time, which
can be precisely calculated in advance.

"The trouble is," John said, "that you ought to have
lymph nodes in the glands in your armpits, for example,
if you had a lymphoma, and you don't. If you had a dysproteinemia you ought to have an abnormal protein in your
urine or blood, and perhaps an enlarged liver and spleen,
and again you don't."

The result of all this "great argument about it and
about" was a nasty shock I found in store for me. It had
been decided, John said, to give me not only a routine
marrow test but a very thorough biopsy. So John first went
into my backbone with the needle and then got out the
sharp miniature sugar tongs he uses for biopsies. He had an
awful time getting the prongs through my backbone, and
by the time he had enough of me in his test tube, he was
sweating. So was I.

As usual, after the thing was done and the holes in my
back had been bandaged up, we chatted.

"Suppose," I asked, "I had a series of normal blood
tests and marrow tests, and these and the biopsies

175

showed no evidence of cancer. Would you at some point pronounce me cured and tell me to go on about my business?"

"No, we won't pronounce you cured as long as we don't know what was wrong with you in the first place. We might keep you under observation for ten years or more, with a blood test every few weeks and a marrow test every six months or so. But whatever happens, it's not going to be like three months ago when you were under a sword of Damocles all the time."

"You mean the sword will be held up, not by a single human hair, but by a fairly dependable rope?"

"Exactly."

We chatted briefly about Bill Gray, who had worked for *Newsweek* and who had been cured at NIH of Hodgkin's disease, a lymph cancer.

"Aside from your having no lymph nodes I can find," John said, "one reason I really don't think you can have a lymphoma is that you have your appetite back and you're feeling fine. You ask your friend Bill Gray how he was feeling when he had a lymphoma—he was feeling God-awful. Also, your night sweats have disappeared."

"Did any of the doctors at the conference have any theory about the night sweats?"

"No. We talked about them. But they're just not typical of leukemia."

"Would you like to hear Dr. Alsop's theory?" (John nods, smiling.) "I think God was wrestling with the Devil every night and finally threw him out of my body."

"That's as good a theory as any we have."

Tish and I go into the waiting area, to join the Nos Morituri Brigade and wait for the blood and marrow results.

176

In the background, as usual, there is the sound of children crying their hearts out—marrow tests hurt, and small veins are hard to find. There are two little boys in the waiting area, patiently reading comic books. Both have the pallor of the leukemic. One is wearing a long black wig, and the other is wearing a shorter blond wig. I scribble in my notebook, "This place has saved my life, but I hate it with all my heart—I suppose because horribilis mors perturbat me."

Then John comes in beaming, and I know the news is good. The blood test readings are all normal, even high normal. "If you'd had these counts when you went to see Dr. Perry in July, he'd have told you you were okay and sent you back to work."

A little later, John called with the results of the marrow test—still less than 6 percent abnormal cells. Later still, he called to say there was not the slightest evidence of lymphoma in the biopsy.

****

On a recent Needwood weekend, brother Joe was very stern with me about this book. It should be an *important* book, he said, and I should make an effort not to write it "in your *Saturday Evening Post* or *Newsweek* style."

Joe is writing an immense work on the history of taste. Reading his book, and then some of what I have written for this book, I can see just what he means. His is indeed an important book, filled with recondite and fascinating information about art and attitudes toward art, about the great collectors of antiquity, about the strange mutations in perceptions of beauty. It is written in a style quite different—more imposing, more marmoreal—than the style in which he writes his columns.

My book is all too obviously written in what he calls my "*Saturday Evening Post* or *Newsweek* style," and it says nothing very important. The reason is that my style is the only style I have, and since I got sick I have discovered nothing very important to say.

I am not a genius and Joe is. Besides being a political journalist, he is an archaeologist manqué, an art critic manqué, a historian manqué, and several other manqué things besides. He switches easily from one role to another. I am a political journalist, period. I have no role to switch to, though I am sometimes tempted to try my hand at a political novel.

IIIIIIIIIIIIIIIIIIIIIIIIIIIIIIIIIIIIIIIIIIIIIIIIIIIIIIIIIIIIIIIIIIIIIIIIIIIIIII

Tuesday, November 30—

After I had published my two *Newsweek* columns on leukemia, I got a surprising number of letters advising me to get in touch with Dr. Isaac Djerassi of Philadelphia. The letter writers had an almost religious faith in his curative powers. My son Joe wrote him first, and then he and I corresponded. Last week I got a letter from him to say that he was coming to Washington today, to visit NIH. I had a date for a blood test at NIH at 2:30, and I suggested that he and Tish and I have lunch and then I would chauffeur him to NIH.

He turned out to be a fascinating fellow—a Bulgarian Jew who had emigrated from Bulgaria to Israel and then here. He is short, with long brown wavy hair, brown expressive eyes, and a mobile, intelligent face. First, briefly, we discussed my case. Like everyone else, he was mystified.

"The blasts in the marrow, yes," he said. "Forty percent abnormal blasts. For those blasts there is no good explanation." The implication—if these abnormal cells were not malignant, what were they doing in the marrow?

Over lunch he described his rather Rube Goldbergian filtration techniques to separate white blood cells from a donor's blood, and he showed pictures of the technique in operation. He is perfectly convinced that he has conquered, or very nearly conquered, the intractable problem of leukocyte transfusion. If he has done so, it will mean not a cancer cure but one of those major advances which taken all together may one day amount to a way of controlling cancer.

Leukocytes are white blood cells. It is their job, and especially the job of the granulocytes, to fight off infections or other alien threats to the body's health—including cancer itself. When a healthy person cuts himself, he will see white pus collecting around the wound. The pus is white blood cells—*pus bonum et laudabile,* the ancients called it—and the cells have been summoned to fight infection.

Way back at the turn of the century, the first blood transfusions were performed, and they have saved tens of thousands of lives since. Platelet transfusions are much more recent; they only began to be successfully performed around the early sixties, and the successful matching of platelets (which is as important as the matching of blood) dates from the late sixties and early seventies. Leukocyte transfusions are very risky, very rare, and used only *in extremis.* This is because the white cells have the shortest half-life of all the three kinds of cells in the blood and are much more likely to be rejected, sometimes violently and dangerously, by the existing white cells.

I am in no position, of course, to judge Dr. Djerassi's

179

experiments. But I telephoned Ed Henderson and Dr. Sidney Farber of Children's Hospital in Boston, and both of them agreed that Djerassi's experiments were of real importance. They also gave him credit for a lot of the new platelet transfusion techniques.

Dr. Henderson says that Djerassi has an unquestioned genius for infuriating the NIH bureaucracy, that he often does the right things for the wrong reasons or at least for reasons he can't explain logically, but that he is also a man of extraordinary intuitive qualities and great medical talents. His leukocyte transfusion technique, if it works, will represent a really major advance.

If cancer is to be cured, it is likely to be cured by such advances, little by little, rather than by some sudden, miraculous, total cure that will eliminate all forms of cancer. And yet it is true, as Dr. Djerassi pointed out at lunch, that all cancers have one common denominator—they all involve the uncontrolled proliferation of abnormal cells. If and when someone discovers what causes them to proliferate—or rather, perhaps, what element in a healthy body prevents them from proliferating—then there could be a "cure" for cancer. Last year at this time I would not have known or cared about Dr. Djerassi's leukocyte transfusion experiments; now they seem to me genuinely exciting. Experience is a great, if painful, teacher.

I drove Dr. Djerassi to NIH, hoping to introduce him to John Glick, but his appointment was in another building. I had a finger stick and then chatted with John Glick for a few minutes while waiting for the results. John speculated about the phenomenon of "smoldering acute leukemia"—a leukemia which lies dormant for some time, then suddenly fulminates. But he added, to my relief, that in my case "nothing fits, no blasts in the peripheral blood, two marrows essentially normal—you really can't have acute leukemia."

180

We again discussed what he calls "the variables": the Atromid, the flu, and, always, allopurinol. I reminded him of a magic copper bracelet, to guard against tennis elbow, which I took off during my first stay at NIH. It really did seem to help my elbow, but it was just after I'd first put it on in London that I got so sick in Paris. Perhaps those greenish patches it leaves around the wrist really do produce a chemical reaction, I suggested, but John was highly skeptical.

"Then how about the Queen Bee Jelly?" I asked. "I swear I began to feel a lot better as soon as I started it."

"Yes," said John, "but your count was going up well before you began on the bee jelly. Sorry, I'm afraid the jelly's out."

"Well, then," I said, "there's one variable you keep leaving out."

"What's that?"

"God," I said.

"That's right," he said.

We both smiled. I don't really believe in God, or at least I don't think I do, and I doubt if John Glick does, but I think we both had at the back of our minds the irrational notion that God might have had something to do with what happened all the same.

Later John telephoned to tell me the blood counts. They are the best yet. "You have the blood of a perfectly normal man," John said.

Thank you God, thank you Mother, thank you Father, thank you Aggie.

P.S. December 3rd. Thank you also, Dr. Djerassi. I picked up the *New York Times* Wednesday to find that Tom Wicker had written the same column I had written, about Nixon and his encounter with the labor bosses—same organization, same conclusion, everything. One of the nastier haz-

181

ards of the column-writing trade. So I tore up the labor piece and made Dr. Djerassi into a column. Not bad, either.

Wednesday, December 15—

At ten thirty I went to NIH to have a marrow test, a blood test, and a physical going over. The marrow wasn't bad—no fun, as usual, but much less painful than the last time.

John took some extra blood out of me, for a lady doctor who wanted to test my blood for some outré disease with a very long name. Because my case is so "bizarre"—the word of art at NIH—I am, as John says, "the most overtested patient in history." As he was taking out my blood and afterward, as he did the routine thumping and feeling and listening, we talked, as usual. Like Dr. Henderson, John is now quite sure I didn't have acute leukemia—I couldn't have had the disease and still be alive without chemotherapy.

I left NIH for the office feeling rather euphoric. It is always a relief to get a marrow test over and done with; the feeling is a bit like getting your feet on the ground after a parachute jump. And I felt so well that I was convinced my troubles were over.

John called at about three, and my euphoria died.

He has a very readable voice, and I could read right away that he was not happy with the results of the tests. The platelets and hemoglobin were holding up, he said, but there had been a rather sharp drop in the granulocyte count. What was more worrying was that the abnormal cells, on a first quick count, had increased by about 50 percent—from the area of 5 percent to 6 percent to around 8 percent to 9 percent. When John said this, my heart sank. Oh, God, here we go again, I thought. I asked him what he thought these results might mean.

"I have to start by saying that I just don't know," he said. "None of us know. But if I had to put my money down, I'd say that allopurinol played a role in your case, but that something else is going on, we don't know what. Whatever it is, it's not galloping. Whatever you have, it may declare itself one day, maybe tomorrow, maybe five years from now."

"Maybe never?" I asked hopefully.

"That's right, maybe never," he said. "All we know is, those bad cells haven't gone away."

"I don't like the growth in the bad cells, John," I said.

"I don't either," he said. "We'll just have to wait and see. I'll test your blood two weeks from today, and if something looks wrong I'll marrow you again. Otherwise, we'll have another marrow a month from now."

For the rest of the afternoon I worked on the column, telephoning various people and typing away. But always in the back of my mind was a small pea of doubt and fear. The pea of doubt was especially disagreeable because in my euphoria I had anticipated what I so much wanted to hear: "Your marrow is normal, and so is your blood. We'll keep an eye on you, but I think you can call yourself cured."

I now suspect I will never hear those welcome words, and that I'll just have to get used to uncertainty. But then, anyone over fifty-five, say, has to live with uncertainty—it is the age when the funerals of friends begin.

Friday, December 17—

John Glick called in the morning and said he was unhappy about our telephone conversation and wanted to talk with Tish and myself face to face. I suggested lunch at the house, and we met there at 12:30.

John came in beaming. He had spent one hour that morning comparing my latest marrow slides with the slides

183

of the two previous marrows, and he had concluded that there really was no essential change. As for the lower white blood count, that was easily explained by the low-grade virus that had been giving me mild stomach problems. It was all over Washington, he said—he'd had it for a couple of weeks himself. A virus lowered the counts, while an infection raised them, so the dip in the counts was perfectly consistent with a virus, and I had plenty of granulocytes to handle the problem.

He'd looked, he said, not only at the abnormal cell count but at the other characteristics of my marrow. A marrow in relapse would show a tendency to "clump"—there would be thick clusters of cells and big empty spaces. My marrow had no clumping tendency. The "cellularity" was normal. A leukemic would tend to be either hypercellular or hypocellular (as I had been in the first two months), but now I was normal.

"There's no doubt about it. Your original marrows looked malignant—those cells were really ugly," John said. "We've shown those marrows to doctors all over the world, and every one of them agrees. But now? I'll say it again. We just don't know. You may hold steady at this level in your marrow for months, maybe for years. You may be run over by a truck at seventy-seven—or you may not. We'll just have to wait and see."

We began talking about the emotional aspects of this kind of situation. I told him what he probably knew, that I had considered taking to Shakespeare's bare bodkin earlier, when things looked really bad, rather than go into chemotherapy (though in retrospect I think I would have taken my chances with chemotherapy). But now, I told John, if things went really wrong, I felt pretty sure I'd resort to the bare bodkin, in the shape of a bottle of sleeping pills.

He didn't seem surprised. Neither was Tish. Actually, I'm not sure what I would do if it turned out I had acute leukemia, after all, and had to choose between chemotherapy and sleeping pills. I think I'd choose the pills, but when you're near death you grasp for life. Perhaps I'd simply refuse to take chemotherapy and then let nature, in the shape of infection, take its course.

I was touched when John said, as he was about to leave, that he had been so worried about that first reading of the marrow that he had had stomach cramps and slept badly. Doctors are people too.

||||||||||||||||||||||||||||||||||||||||||||||||||||||||||||||||||||||||||||||||

Ian and his friend Jill Charlton are back from Katmandu, and the house is rapidly filling up for Christmas with the other children. Ian looks dashing, if somewhat piebald. He has light blond hair, jet black eyebrows, blue eyes, a brown moustache, and a dark auburn beard, grown after the fashion of Nicolai Lenin. Tish and I had been a bit nervous about meeting Jill. Ian got to know her on the Far Eastern youth circuit, in New Delhi, where much hash is smoked and many pills popped, and we didn't know what to expect.

She turns out to be a small, charming girl, sensible and practical, with a tendency to wear dresses (if that is what they are called) that come down to her ankles, so that she looks like an illustration from *Punch,* circa 1880. She reminds me oddly of Sis at the same age—she has the same authoritative, no-nonsense air. Her favorite word is the adjective "fantastic," with the accent heavily on the second

185

syllable. It is used for all forms of approval. It is oddly catching; we have all begun describing things as "fan*tas*tic." The word even crept into a recent column, before I caught it and expunged it.

About a year after I'd said good-bye to Ian at the Hotel Caravelle in Saigon just before Christmas 1969, I wrote him one of those parental letters. Part of the letter was about the importance of hanging onto capital; Ian had spent a couple of thousand of the limited number of dollars he had inherited. My thesis was that having a bit of capital, even a few thousand dollars, gives a man a certain independence, an ability to thumb his nose at other men. This part of my letter Ian took in good part, I think—as to all Alsops, independence is very dear to him. But then I couldn't forebear to add one of those snotty parental wisecracks:

"As for the longer future, I think you must ask yourself whether you really want to spend the rest of your life as a Nepalese woodcut peddler."

This irritated Ian, as he has since made clear, and I confess I think he was right to be irritated. When I wrote the letter, he and Jill had just invented their unique business, which they have since greatly expanded. When the Communists moved into Tibet in 1959, the Dalai Lama and his priesthood moved out, mostly into Nepal. They brought with them, as well as many ancient artifacts, hundreds of traditional woodcuts, finely carved, from which black and white engravings with religious or symbolic motifs are made on rice paper.

Ian and Jill acquired some woodcuts and began selling the rice-paper prints on the streets of Katmandu, one of several fashionable Far Eastern gathering places for the liberated young. This venture, it seems, had a fan*tas*tic success, to the point where Ian and Jill have two Nepalese

186

permamently employed, helping them turn out the prints, which is hard work. They also have a house, decorated with prints and artifacts and boasting a flush toilet, one of the few in Katmandu. They intend to take a water-bed back with them to Katmandu, for a final touch of comfort. Their purpose in coming here, aside from seeing the family, was to hold an exhibition of Tibetan prints in Georgetown and to try to start a print-exporting business to the United States.

Ian brought me as a present a small martial god, made of very coppery brass and brandishing a sword. I like it very much and have it prominently displayed in my dressing room. The prints, I confess, are not my sort of thing; they are too busy and one-dimensional for my eye, and they symbolize meanings which I do not begin to understand. A matter of education of the taste, I suppose—brother Joe, whose taste is educated in such matters, finds some of them beautiful.

In any case, Ian is serious about the prints and the artifacts and very knowledgeable about them; he is well on the way to becoming a true expert in the rather arcane field of Himalayan art. As for his being a Nepalese woodcut peddler, he is a very successful Nepalese woodcut peddler. He and Jill live well, and he has not dipped into his small store of capital in a long time. Katmandu, it appears, is a lovely place—smiling people and eternal spring. So why shouldn't he remain a Nepalese woodcut peddler as long as he chooses?

The Alsops made their money peddling rum in the West Indies and maybe a bit of opium in the China trade. I suppose peddling woodcuts is as respectable a form of peddling, and maybe more so.

Ian went through a period in Dartmouth when he lived

on LSD, hash, and tiny portions of rice permitted him under some sort of Zen Buddhist diet. He looked as though a light wind would blow him away, but meanwhile he was making Phi Beta Kappa in junior year, which as far as I know no other Alsop has ever done. There was a period, fortunately brief, when he would wander about the house, looking famished and smiling a curiously vacuous smile. This, we learned subsequently, was "the smile of inner benignity" which Zen Buddhists wear as an armor against the slings and arrows of outrageous squaredom.

The smile of inner benignity drove Tish and myself up the wall, but except for that brief period, Ian has always been excellent company—witty, a good mimic, and with a curious basic innocence, a lack of sham and *arrière pensée* which is, I think, indestructible, and the secret of his charm.

Joe and Candy have arrived, and Joe is very critical of my handling, if it can be called handling, of Nicky and Andrew. "Daddy," he will say, when one or the other is defying my feeble will or making himself obnoxious in some way, "how can you let them get away with that?"

The truth is that I am a weakly permissive parent, but it is also true, as I explained to him the other day, that this is partly Joe's fault. When Joe was about Andrew's age, he had a passion for toy trucks. He learned to talk before he was four, but until he was about six, he retained an oddity of speech—the sound of the letters "tr" he pronounced as if they formed an "f." This led to a major embarrassment.

Tish and I, egged on to do so by brother Joe, who considers giving dinner parties part of a columnist's job, gave a large, pompous dinner party in 1949 in our Dumbarton Avenue house. (Brother Joe is right, but I have always been lazy about this part of a columnist's job—I like being a guest, but I much dislike being a host.) Cousin Alice Longworth was a guest, and so was the British Ambassador of the era (then a very important person in Washington), and there were a couple of Senators, fellow columnists, and the like.

As the guests began to arrive, I told "little Joe" (now six foot three) to collect his toys and go on up to bed. Children have an animal instinct about these things. He sensed that this would be a good time to test my will, and he went on playing with his toy trucks on the living room floor. He was still there when the last guest had arrived. I told Joe to go to bed, in my best this-time-goddammit-I-mean-it tone. He went on playing with his trucks.

I knew that it was now or never and grabbed him around the waist, while a hush fell on the party. In that house, the stairs leading to the second floor bedrooms were open stairs, in the living room. By the time we got to the stairs, Joe was kicking like a mule and howling like a banshee. On the way up, he grabbed a banister, hung on for dear life, and began to shout a nonnegotiable demand: "Give me my little trucks! Give me my little trucks!"

Only that was not quite what he said. As usual, he pronounced "tr" with the sound "f." I succeeded in loosening his hold on the banister and got him halfway up the stairs. He grabbed another banister and continued to shout his nonnegotiable demand.

At this point Tish gathered up the toy trucks and came up the stairs, briskly and threateningly. Joe released his hold on the banister. Tish administered a hard, no-nonsense spanking and put him to bed, while I went downstairs and tried to make conversation as though nothing had happened. Nobody said anything about the incident; in those days, the word that Joe had been shouting was *never* used in respectable mixed company. But I think several of the guests,

189

Cousin Alice especially, were secretly amused.

This episode enfeebled further my already dubious authority over little Joe and encouraged my tendency to play the role of permissive parent and leave discipline up to Tish. Sometimes, when driven too far, I would break into a sudden purple-faced rage—I still do, when Andrew or Nicky gets on my nerves. But by and large I am easygoing old Daddy, and all the children in turn have sensed that the parent to take seriously is Tish.

I am rather surprised that Joe is so deeply irritated by my tendency to let Nicky and Andrew get away with their various outrages. Perhaps there is something generational at work here. Father was very much paterfamilias and expected his word to be obeyed without question. Joe and John and I all went through a period when we seethed with rebellion against Pa, especially when we were dependent on him financially. I am perhaps too permissive with my children because I remember too vividly how bitterly I used to resent Pa's authoritarian ways.

In my day, antiparental rebellion took the form of drinking too much in college and at debutante parties, driving too fast, and getting involved with "unsuitable" girls. Sooner or later, of course, the rebel got into trouble. I got into trouble in sophomore year in college.

I shared a Model-A Ford touring car with brother John; with sophomoric humor we called it "Artur Arturinka." A friend called Bob McCormick and I (Where are you now, Bob? Haven't seen you in twenty years) dropped in one night at an establishment called the York Athletic Club, New Haven's leading speakeasy, which went on behaving like a speakeasy even after Prohibition was repealed. At the York A.C. we met two young ladies. We suggested that we drive to Bridgeport in search of adventure, the girls agreed,

190

and we climbed into Artur Arturinka. One of the girls sat up front with me, and the other one, whose name was Carla Scarletti, sat on Bob McCormick's lap in the back of the open Ford. I drove too fast, of course—I had been drinking bathtub gin and ginger ale at the York Athletic Club—and when I passed a truck and just barely missed it, poor Carla began to scream. Her arm had been draped over the side of the touring car, and the truck had scraped it.

We turned around and took Carla to the New Haven Hospital. Carla's two enormous brothers arrived, and we heard them asking for the names of the "Yale college punks" and threatening to "sue the bejesus out of them." The hospital desk gave them our names, while Bob and I scuttled out of the place and back to the sanctuary of Yale.

When I woke up the next morning, I knew what I had to do. I had to call Pa. I went to classes, and then I went to the fraternity bar and had two old-fashioneds and called Pa's office in Hartford. When he came on the telephone, the conversation that ensued was brief.

"Father," I said (for this was too serious an occasion to call him Pa), "I'm in trouble."

"Oh, God, Stewart," he said. "What's her name?"

"Carla Scarletti, Father," I said.

"Oh, Jesus Christ," he said, and hung up the telephone.

Afterward, Father was quite nice about the whole episode, even though the automobile insurance rates he had to pay were almost doubled. I think he was relieved that he had misjudged the kind of trouble I was in.

This small episode from my not very bright college days has a curiously musty air. Yale was very Waspish and establishmentarian in those days, of course. Rebellion was not limited to drinking and driving too fast. It also took a political form. Most of my politically minded friends were left-

191

liberal New Dealers, and a good many were, like myself, at least theoretical Marxists. But there were limits to rebellion. Among all my rebellious friends, I know of none who lived openly with a girl while not in a state of matrimony; a love affair in those days was a much more hole-in-corner business than it is today. Times have changed.

But times change only up to a point. Drink and fast driving and conventional Marxism have been replaced as symbols of rebellion by pot and long hair and public cohabitation and a strange variety of revolutionary doctrines. When Joe and Candy have children, and their children get to the age where they worry about pimples and resent their parents, rebellion will take some different form, but rebellion there will be. If they have boys, I think I can confidently predict that the boys will rebel with special fury against son Joe, just because Joe has the kind of strong character male children always rebel against. I hope Candy can cope. I think she can, because she has, despite a pretty face and gentle manner, as strong a character as Joe—maybe stronger.

When Joe graduated from M.I.T. in 1969, he announced that he intended to be "independently wealthy" by the time he was thirty. Asked to define the term, he said it meant a million dollars in capital at a minimum, but preferably ten million, which should not be too difficult. Intercomp—International Computation, Inc.—was to be the initial vehicle of his independence. Intercomp, which Joe helped found, makes a "widget" called an "interface." The interface, as I imperfectly understand it, transforms one of the cheaper IBM machines into the equivalent of a much more expensive IBM machine, and it sells, or leases, for much less than the difference.

In my simple-minded way, I spotted the essential weak-

192

ness of Intercomp at the start. I asked Joe if the widget could be protected by patent. Joe said he had looked into that, and it couldn't. It was, he explained, "just an idea, as though you had the idea of making a table by putting four legs on a door," and this kind of idea could not be patented. A few weeks ago, the inevitable happened. IBM began to make its own widget, cheaper and better serviced than the Intercomp widget. There is a line in Pope about breaking a butterfly upon a wheel. In this case, the butterfly was Intercomp, and IBM the wheel.

All three Alsop brothers put a bit of capital into Intercomp. I was reluctant, being cautious by nature, but something my brother John said persuaded me. "Stew," he said, "if you don't invest in Intercomp, in a few years people will be saying, 'Why isn't that Stewart Alsop one of the rich Alsops? All the other Alsops are rich, and yet he's the father of that Intercomp genius, isn't he?'" Naturally, this remark aroused all my sibling rivalry, and I sold some insurance stock (which has since done well) to put the money into Intercomp. Since IBM made its butterfly-breaking move, our investment does not look very brilliant.

Son Joe is undaunted, though. He is not easily dauntable. In fact he is mule-stubborn, as he proved that night with his little trucks, as well as very able, and although he may not be "independently wealthy" at thirty, I think he will be a genuinely successful man sooner or later. Maybe he is a genuinely successful man already. He is busy, deeply interested in what he is doing, healthy, and happily married. It is hard to think of a better definition of success.

Elizabeth—Fuff—and her husband, Peter Mahony, are here, and the house is bursting at the seams. Fuff is mule-stubborn too. She is so stubborn that, as a fellow-professional writer, I am filled with admiration. Fuff works at Harper &

193

Row, in the children's book department, and Peter works with an up-and-coming New York architectural firm, where he specializes in urban planning and is doing, I gather, extremely well.

Peter is a handsome young man. With his mustache and his wavy brown hair, he looks a bit like the kind of young man Charles Dana Gibson used to draw, wooing one of his Gibson girls. Fuff is attractive, but she does not look like a Gibson girl. For one thing, she has too firm a jaw. Peter first started wooing Fuff when she was fifteen, and Tish and I used to worry that Fuff, stubborn as she is, would dominate Peter. We worry no longer. Fuff used to swear that never, never, never would she live in New York City. When Peter got a promising job offer from the New York architectural firm, she dug in her heels and ululated. I quoted Ruth in the Bible to her—"Whither thou goest, I will go; and where thou lodgest, I will lodge"—and she dug in her heels and ululated louder. Peter said nothing. Now they are sharing an apartment in Gramercy Park in Manhattan.

The apartment consists of a room just big enough to get a double bed into, another room in which it would be difficult to swing a full-grown cat, and a closet which, when opened, turns out to harbor a tiny stove and a tinier refrigerator. For $325 a month, God help us.

With my claustrophobia, I find it mysterious that any marriage could survive life in a box. But that is not all. Every night, after she comes home from work and makes their supper, Fuff sits stubbornly down at a typewriter and starts tapping away. She is a professional writer, what is more—a writer who gets paid for what she writes.

She has had several short stories published in somewhat obscure literary magazines. Harper's has accepted a children's book by her called *Bunk Beds,* and she is at work on a

194

novel for teen-agers called *Walking Away*. (I thought that teen-agers didn't read any more, but apparently there is a big market for teen-age fiction.) Fuff's characters tend to be somewhat recognizable. *Bunk Beds,* for example, is about Ian and Fuff and the bunk beds they shared when they were very small and we lived on Dumbarton Avenue. Nicky has inherited the bunk beds, and sometimes, as a high honor, he lets Andrew sleep in the top bed.

Walking Away is about Emily, a girl who goes to visit her grandfather and grandmother on a farm in Virginia. Emily invites a sophisticated girl friend to the farm, and the girl friend comes between Emily and Grandfather, who had been close. The farm is markedly like Polecat Park, right down to the sagging cement porch and the lilac bush outside the kitchen window. Emily is a Fufflike girl, and the friend is like a pretty blonde Fuff used to invite to Polecat Park. As for Grandfather, he has certain peculiar characteristics—peculiar to me.

Ever since Fuff was a little girl, I have been sewing up one or another of my three Aubusson rugs with a curved needle, sitting cross-legged on the floor. I have a passion for Aubusson rugs, and if you own Aubussons, unless you want to spend thousands a year having them repaired, you learn to use the curved needle. In *Walking Away*, Emily and her girl friend come into the farmhouse one evening, and there is Grandfather, squatting on the floor and sewing up his rug.

At Polecat Park, I invented a restful way of fishing. I would take an inner tube down to the pond, and put my bottom in the hole, and propel myself with my feet, and use my fly rod to cast into the otherwise inaccessible parts of the pond. In *Walking Away*, Emily comes upon dear old Grandpa, fly-fishing for bass, with his bottom in an inner tube.

195

Grandfather emerges as a likable old fellow but a some-what atypical Virginia dirt farmer. He dies in the end, of course, and there's not a dry eye in the house.

In fact, Fuff has real talent, as well as an awesome determination to become a serious writer. The combination can hardly fail to pay off in the end. But as I've told her, sometimes I worry that she'll run out of family and friends before her talent comes to full flower.

Stewart, nineteen and a freshman at Occidental College in Los Angeles, also has aspirations as a writer. He is currently at work on a long short story about his life at Groton. His style is markedly baroque, with many similes ("My head felt like a pail full of dirty water"), in contrast to Fuff's style, which is rather Plain Jane. But he shares with Fuff a certain recognizability in his characters. The frightened little boy who is deposited at boarding school by his parents has a mother who "has no personal vanity at all" and who, when she bends down to pick something up, never bends her knees—both very recognizable characteristics of Tish. The boy's father has a pink face, a big nose, brushes his hair straight back, and has, rather surprisingly, "clawlike hands."

I read Stewart's story with fascination, because I was once myself a frightened little boy deposited at boarding school by his parents. I disliked Groton very much, especially at first, and was constantly getting into trouble there. I got into especially bad trouble in Fifth Form year, trying to get out of trouble. The initial trouble I had got into—I've forgotten what it was, exactly—was bad enough so that Dr. Peabody had told Father he was thinking of expelling me when the term ended. Brother Joe suggested that the best way to strengthen my defenses was to tell Dr. Peabody that I wanted to be confirmed, since this was sure to please him. I did so and duly appeared at a series of religious talks Dr.

Peabody gave in the evenings in his study (the same study son Joe later bugged) for the boys who were to be confirmed.

A few days before my confirmation was to take place, I was summoned to the rector's study and found myself alone with the great man. Previously, every time I had been alone with Dr. Peabody, I had been in some sort of bad trouble. Dr. Peabody had a curiously hypnotic effect on a lot of boys, including myself, and I felt a mental catatonia creeping over me.

Dr. Peabody talked at some length, presumably about religion—I was too catatonic to listen—when he suddenly interrupted himself with a question: "Tell me, boy, to what denomination do you belong?"

The question must have been asked with malice aforethought. Groton was a church school, and almost everyone who went there was an Episcopalian. Dr. Peabody must have know that my father and all my other numerous Groton relations were Episcopalians. At any rate, at this point, my mental catatonia became total. It was as though a dark curtain had been drawn over my brain. I couldn't remember the word "Episcopalian."

I felt a mounting panic. Having applied for confirmation, I couldn't possibly tell Dr. Peabody that I didn't know to what denomination I belonged. As it happened, I shared a study that year with Huston Huffman, a Baptist, the only Baptist in the school. The word "Baptist" popped into my mind.

"I am a Baptist, sir," I said.

"A Baptist?" said Dr. Peabody, in what I now suspect was feigned surprise. "That is odd. I was quite sure your father was an Episcopalian. However . . ."

After the interview, Dr. Peabody telephoned Father, told him I had apparently been converted to Baptism, and suggested that a total immersion seemed appropriate. Father

197

had to race up to Groton in his Stutz Bearcat to rescue me, as he had done at least twice before. I think now the whole painful episode was Dr. Peabody's way of letting it be known that he wasn't fooled by my sudden religious conversion. But he didn't expel me after all, and like Joe and John, I graduated from Groton with a proper diploma to prove it.

Only one of my three oldest boys—Ian—graduated from Groton, and all three hated the place. My mother and a lot of other people were furious at Dr. Crocker, Dr. Peabody's successor, for expelling Joe for bugging his study, but I could not argue with conviction against Dr. Crocker's decision. For one thing, invasion of privacy is a serious matter. For another, if a boy had bugged Dr. Peabody's study, the boy would not have been fired. He would have been immolated by a thunderbolt sent direct from heaven on Dr. Peabody's orders.

The study bugging was only one of a number of operations mounted by Joe and a small band of classmates. In another operation, the clock on the chapel tower, which regulated the whole Groton day with its chimes, was set back, so that everybody got up late, ate breakfast late, went to classes late, and so on. Joe was expelled in 1963—pre-Vietnam, pre-long hair, pre-pot. So this was the familiar phenomenon of generational rebellion. But it was rebellion on a greater scale, and far more daring, than anything imaginable in my era at Groton.

Ian, one gathers, floated through Groton rather like a disembodied spirit. He got a good education, which stood him in good stead at Dartmouth, but otherwise he was at Groton only in body, never in spirit. He made no lasting friendships, took no part in extracurricular activities. He just survived, like the Abbé Sieyès, and waited for liberation.

Stewart, more than Joe or Ian, really hated Groton. The quality of his hatred of the place comes out clearly in his story, "The Magic Forest." He felt suffocated by the school. When the sense of suffocation became unbearable, he would escape to the "magic forest," the woods that surround the school. Unlike Joe, Stewart wasn't expelled. He could have graduated, but by the end of his Fifth Form year—one year before graduation—it was clear to Tish and myself that in some mysterious way Groton was hurting Stewart badly. We pulled him out and sent him to Suffield, where Joe had gone after he was expelled, and where Stewart was much less unhappy.

In my generation, my younger brother John actually enjoyed Groton—he was popular, editor-in-chief of the *Grotonian*, on the football team, and in Sixth Form year he was made a prefect, the ultimate honor. Joe and I disliked the place. Joe was regarded as more eccentric than I was, but I got into more trouble than he did. But both of us became involved in the school—we made friends, some of whom are still friends, and we were both editors of the *Grotonian* and members of the Drama Society, and the like.

All three of my boys seem to have decided, in their different ways, that the school was the Enemy, and they either fought it or had as little to do with it as possible. Why? A difference in them? In the school? In the times? I don't know. I think we were somehow conditioned to accept a degree of misery and discomfort—hard discipline, cold showers only, bad food, no girls,—that our children's generation is unwilling and unprepared to accept. In any case, while Groton was a net plus for Joe and John and myself, it was clearly a net minus for Joe and Ian and Stewart. Neither Nicky nor Andrew will go to Groton.

Stewart was much the handsomest of the children when he was a little boy. He was always cheerful, and not so long ago I especially enjoyed dandling him on my knee. He is now enormous—as tall as Joe and over 200 pounds. If I tried

199

to dandle him on my knee, I would be broken like a butterfly, as Intercomp was broken by IBM. But he is still cheerful and good company, and when he is older and cuts off some of his Afro, he will again be the handsomest of the children. I think he can write; allowing for the prejudices of a parent who had a similar experience long ago, I find "The Magic Forest" moving. If he can tame his baroque style and achieve some of Fuff's stubborn self-discipline, Stewart might write really well.

I have always had a perhaps unhealthy obsession with my youngest child. I adored first Joe, then Ian, then Elizabeth, then Stewart. I didn't adore them when they were babies—babies have always seemed to me singularly boring human beings, if that is what they are. I began to adore them when they were just turning into real human beings, at about two. I began to stop adoring them at about seven or eight. That is when knee-dandling becomes impractical. It is also the beginning of the end of innocence, the beginning of growing up. It is when a child's eyes become a little guarded, turn a bit opaque, and the child ceases, little by little, to be a child.

My obsession with Nicky, who was a postscript, seven years after Stewart, was especially powerful. This was partly because when he was very young Nicky was a rather sickly little boy, with a wandering eye. We tried to keep a patch over his good eye, so that the bad eye would catch up, but it didn't work. Finally Nicky had an operation, which brought both eyes into line, but the bad eye had, and still has, only faint peripheral vision. Because of his eye trouble, Nicky had great trouble learning to read and write. This aroused my protective instincts and made me more permissive than ever.

Nicky is twelve now, and it is already clear that he is

going to be even more enormous than Joe and Stewart. It is also clear that, being a determined fellow, he is going to be able to read and write properly, though the struggle has not been easy for him. He is getting to the age where his voice sometimes sounds like the cry of an adolescent alligator in rut, and he can still arouse me to occasional purple-faced paroxysms. There are signs of the inevitable rebellion on the way, and I no longer have an unhealthy obsession about him. But he is full of vitality, and fun to be with, and I have much affection for him. When he is not in full revolt, we are friends.

My unhealthy obsession has been transferred to Andrew, who is almost five and a sort of post-postscript, or do-it-yourself grandson, as Tish says. Andrew is a good-looking little boy—almost as good-looking as Stewart at his age—and he has a wide, rather cynical grin, which displays a missing tooth right in the middle of his mouth. He invariably amuses me and cheers me up. I may be a foolish fond old man, but I even claim to discern in some of his remarks something very like conscious wit. For example, Stewart brought a pretty, tall, willowy girl friend home. As she sashayed through the living room, Andrew remarked, "I like the way she wiggles her things."

But the time is coming fairly soon when knee-dandling will be impractical for Andrew too. There will be no post-post-postscript. So I wish the older children would get busy and supply us with some knee-dandlers with unguarded eyes.

All this sounds a bit smarmy-sentimental, but then advancing age and a serious illness make a man sentimental. Moreover, after I get over my initial obsession, I am not at all sentimental about the children, and neither is Tish. In fact, we shove them out of the nest as soon as they can flutter their wings, and although we like to have them about for holidays and weekends and the like, they are on their own.

As a result we are all, I think, despite inevitable conflicts, friends who lead their own lives. This is the best relationship between parents and children. A neurotic emotional interdependence between parents and children, above all between mothers and sons, has, I suspect, wrecked more lives than all history's wars.

The subject of my disease has hardly been mentioned between the children and myself. The line now is that "Daddy's much better," and the children and I leave it at that. As this suggests, there is a certain arm's-length relationship between us, a fear on both sides of invading the other side's privacy. To me, this seems a healthy relationship.

||||||||||||||||||||||||||||||||||||||||||||||||||||||||||||||||||||||||||||||

Wednesday, December 29, 1971—

Isaac Djerassi called on Monday and said that, since I wrote my column about him, he felt a "personal responsibility" toward me. So he wanted to see my marrow slides and, if he saw what he expected, urge my doctor to use a vaccine on me called BCG. The vaccine was originally developed for use against tuberculosis, but it has been found by a group headed by a Dr. Mathé in Paris to have an immunizing effect against leukemia.

I asked him when he was coming to Washington, and he said he had an appointment at NIH on January 21, so I suggested that we get together with John Glick then.

"No," he said. "We should not lose a day. If immunization is called for, better it was done yesterday."

He has a heavy Bulgarian accent, and everything he says sounds like an actor imitating a man speaking with a heavy Bulgarian accent.

So I told him that I had a blood test at ten thirty on Wednesday, and maybe he'd like to get together with John Glick then to look at the slides. "Okay," he said. "I'll be there." I called Glick, who said he'd be happy to show Djerassi the slides. I called Djerassi, and we agreed to breakfast at his motel near NIH before the blood test.

At breakfast, Djerassi talked about the immunization technique. As I understand it, the technique involves taking your own abnormal cells and injecting them into the skin, with BCG, to stimulate the white cells to attack them. Thus when there is a relapse, the lymphocytes are all primed and eager to do battle. No doubt this is an oversimplification, but it was what I gathered through a lot of technical talk overlaid with a Bulgarian accent.

After breakfast, Tish and I drove Dr. Djerassi over to the clinic at NIH and introduced him to John Glick. They look very different but have something in common, a sort of brilliant intensity. John produced a series of my slides and started with the first NIH slide, with about 40-percent bad cells. Their two heads were bent over the two-sided microscope, an odd unforgettable sight.

"You see these," said Glick, maneuvering the slide with a little wheel. "They look very myeloblastic."

"Yes, they do," said Djerassi.

There was an intercom call for Dr. Glick, and he abandoned the microscope and picked up the telephone.

"Hello. Oh, hello, Fred. Yes, you're going to need some platelets. Your hemoglobin and white count are okay but your platelets are down around sixteen thousand. Yes, three thirty this afternoon—we'll be ready."

Last year, this would have meant nothing to me. Now it meant that poor Fred was in bad trouble. Probably in relapse. Probably a member of the Nos Morituri Brigade. Glick went back to the microscope.

"This is an abnormal plasma cell," said Djerassi, maneuvering the slide.

"Yes."

"I have an auto-immune patient. The dye is not very clear in this slide, but the cell looks very much the same."

Auto-immune? Presumably someone who had leukemia and had developed an immune reaction to it?

Glick: "Here are the cells that looked especially bad to us. They looked very malignant."

Djerassi: "They don't look too good. They look ugly. Very ugly." (Pronounced "varry ogly.")

Glick: "We've shown them to a lot of people, and nobody has ever said they'd like to meet them in a dark alley."

Djerassi: "Looking at these, I'd say you had a stroke of genius not to put him into chemotherapy."

Glick: "Yes, they're very scary, all right, aren't they?"

Then a lot of talk about how the cells are atypical, even though most of them look like myeloblasts. Goddammit, I thought to myself, these are my own private cells inside my own bones they're talking about.

Glick takes out the second-to-last slide, the *dies gloriae* slide, October 11, 6 percent abnormal.

Djerassi looks at it through the microscope, while Glick beams like a fond parent.

Djerassi: "Extraordinary. Even miraculous." (A pause, as he twiddles with the microscope.) "But there are still some blasts left. Are there not?"

John twiddles. "Yes, Stew knows that."

Then some more technical talk, about the absence of "Auer rods" in the blasts. John does a little sketch of a blast for Tish and myself: a small circle within a larger circle, with a line—the Auer rod—that looks like an arrow in the larger circle pointing toward the smaller circle. Auer rods are characteristic of classic AML, so why don't I have them? The obvious answer: I don't have classic AML.

Then what do I have? Both Djerassi and Glick are a bit embarrassed by this question, because doctors like to have answers, and they don't. But after asking both of them separately, I find they have essentially the same answer. Either I have a "smoldering leukemia"—a kind of caged beast, which may break out of its cage at any time or may never break out—or I have no cancer at all. In the latter case, I have simply had a wholly unique and totally idiosyncratic reaction to allopurinol or, if not to allopurinol, to some other unknown factor.

I hope the second answer is correct. Meanwhile, as John says, I'll just have to get used to living with uncertainty.

Finally, the blood-test results come in. Hemoglobin a magnificent 16. "Sixteen is supposed to be normal for a man, fourteen for a woman," says Djerassi, "but hardly anyone is normal. Everybody is more low."

The white blood count is well within normal range. But there is the usual small surprise and mystery: the platelets are sharply down. Why? John Glick says he doesn't know, nobody knows, and it doesn't surprise him especially—platelets are the most wide-ranging of the cell counts.

Good-byes, happy New Years, and we drive Dr. Djerassi back to his motel. In the car he advances a theory that I don't entirely understand. "You think your low platelet count is bad news," he says. "I think it is maybe good news.

Your auto-immune reaction is working to lower the platelets." I gather he thinks the white cells whose job it is to attack an alien body are attacking the platelets, more or less for practice, just to keep their hand in.

Later, when John calls up for a chat before he goes on vacation, I put this theory up to him. He sounds skeptical, to put it mildly. I suspect I got Dr. Djerassi's theory wrong.

Neither of them said so, and Djerassi gave John credit for "genius" for not putting me into chemotherapy despite those "varry ogly" cells, but I sensed they were not at all on the same wave length. Perhaps the reason is that they are different kinds of doctors. Djerassi is essentially a theoretician and, judging by results, a brilliant one. Glick is essentially a physician, in the traditional sense, a man deeply and primarily concerned with saving or prolonging a patient's life. Thank God he is so good at it.

At the end of our telephone chat, John said, "Look, I know you're a bit worried about those platelets—there's always something to worry about. But look at it this way. Last July, I very much doubted that you'd make it to Christmas. Well, you've had a fine Christmas, and you played three sets of tennis yesterday. So count your blessings."

Good advice. But I didn't realize he had taken such a dim view of my prospects. A matter of my age, I suppose. Last July, I myself was hoping to see at least one more spring.

January 10—

Bad news. Into NIH for a blood count. Tish and I met John in the hall, and he asked me how I'd been feeling, and I told him I'd been feeling okay, but not so full of beans as in October and November, when my counts were zooming up. Maybe, I said, it was just psychological, and John agreed; the euphoria of those early days of recovery certainly had something to do with my feeling of physical well-being. But I also had this flulike stomach trouble, I said, a kind of queasiness, and it had lasted for a month. Maybe that had something to do with it too.

I had my finger pricked by the finger-stick lady and went back to the *Newsweek* office. A pleasant lunch with Rowly Evans and Charlie Whitehead—he's going to Saigon as number two. A note to call John when I got back to the office. I didn't have to read John's voice this time.

"We have your counts and I don't like the look of it," he said right away. "Your hemoglobin is fine, but your white blood count and your platelets are both down—the platelets are down to sixty-nine thousand."

"What do you think it means, John?"

"I don't know, but you're leaving Wednesday for Georgia, aren't you? I think we'd better marrow you before you go."

"How about right away?"

"I'll be here, any time you want."

"Okay, I'll pick up Tish and be there in less than an hour." It is better to know than not to know.

I told Amanda that I had to go to NIH to get a marrow test, and she said, "Now, Stew, it's going to be all right." This is always oddly comforting—it is a sort of incantation to which Amanda resorts when things go wrong. I drove back to the house, told Tish, and she called to beg off the dinner party tonight at the British Embassy. Tish has a streaming cold, and we both suspected that we wouldn't be in the mood for a party.

John met me in the hall again. Into a treatment room, with a nurse and a doctor whose name I didn't catch, who

207

is going to try another experiment with my marrow. The experiment is interesting and elaborate, and we discussed it as John went into my back four times—I find it usefully attention-distracting to talk while I'm being marrowed. We had "no spicules" three times in a row, until John finally got out a specimen that was acceptable to both the technician and the experimental doctor. I'm pretty used to it by now—this is my eleventh or twelfth marrow test—but the wait afterward, to let John give us a preliminary reading, was intolerable.

I pretty well knew that the results would be bad, partly because the counts so indicated but mostly because I sensed what John expected. The question was: How bad? Ten percent bad cells? Maybe 30 percent? Tish and I waited in an operating room for what seemed an hour. She read *The Splendid Century*, placidly enough, it seemed, but I don't think she was reading much, and I tried to read *Life* and then went to the bathroom, not because I needed to, but because I couldn't sit still. Then John came in, bad news on his face but not terrible news.

"The proportion of bad cells is definitely up," he said firmly. "They look like about twelve to thirteen percent—certainly between ten and fifteen percent. Whatever happened, it hasn't galloped. But the number of megakaryocytes is definitely down—that accounts for your low platelets. The red cells are excellent. But there's no concealing the fact that this is an obvious setback. You've always been a realist about this, Stew, and you have always realized that there might be more to this than just the allopurinol."

"What does it mean, John?"

"We don't know, of course. But let's suppose you have some unknown malignancy—we don't know you have, but let's suppose you have. This malignancy became very much better. Then something happened to make it worse again. Why? Again, we don't know. Some diseases are cyclic. This is not anything like classic AML. But it could be some form of smoldering leukemia."

"Have there been many cases of smoldering leukemia?"

"No. It's rare—very rare."

"What's the prognosis?"

"It's so rare that you can't make any firm prognosis. But if you have smoldering leukemia, you might live for years. Moreover, you wouldn't have the kind of chemotherapy you would have for AML. We're very aggressive with AML, as you know, but this would be different—a matter of trying to control a disease which was not galloping. You would probably have doses of chemicals on an outpatient basis. But I repeat, we don't know. Suppose your counts go down to six percent or even two percent two months from now. What do we say then? That you're cured? No. That you have some wholly idiosyncratic form of, say, 'cyclic Alsop's disease'? We don't know. All we know is that the bad cells are up and the counts are down, and the two go together."

So what should I do?

John says that I should go to Georgia, as planned, but take it a bit easy—"no traumas." That would be better than "moping about Washington," and meanwhile there's nothing to do but watch the counts.

"This recrudescence has been disturbing to me, and I know it's even more disturbing to you two. You'll be down in the dumps for a while, but you just have to learn to live with this uncertainty."

I ask John again about Djerassi's idea, for an immunological experiment with BCG, the substance Mathé has found effective in inducing a self-immunizing effect in leukemia. John remains wholly skeptical. The technique, he

209

says, has been used at NIH only on children and only for acute lymphoblastic leukemia, which is typically a children's disease. Moreover, it involves injecting blasts, or abnormal cells, from the patient's own marrow along with the BCG, to stimulate the counterattack by the white cells. To get enough blasts from my marrow—since there are not many there—would involve major surgery. Altogether, very dubious.

This "recrudescence" has been a shock to me, but rather less of a shock than I might have expected. I don't know why. I think I've sort of half expected it, ever since the slight increase in the bad cells with the last marrow—that and my seemingly endless stomach problems. I anticipated it, the way the stock market is supposed to anticipate ups and downs, and that has eased the shock a bit. The pea of fear has grown suddenly larger. But it has always been there, at the back of my mind.

Thomasville, Ga.
Monday, January 17—

John Glick gave me a To Whom It May Concern letter to deliver to a doctor in Thomasville, Georgia, where Tish and I are spending a luxurious quail-shooting week with the Jock Whitneys. When we arrived, I remarked half jokingly to Betsey Whitney that parsley was supposed to be good for the blood count. The next morning at breakfast a bowl of chopped parsley appeared beside my plate, and I have had a ration of parsley with every marvelous Whitney meal.

Until yesterday, I had pretty well managed to forget about the recrudescence. There is nothing better than quail shooting for making you forget what you don't want to remember, and since the quail shooting at Greenwood, the

lovely Whitney place here, is the best in the United States—
and thus in the world, for the American bobwhite is a strictly
indigenous bird—that makes the forgetting all the easier.

But yesterday was Sunday, with no shooting. My To
Whom It May Concern letter, which instructed the doctor
to tell me my own blood counts (some doctors are secretive
about such things), had been delivered to a Dr. Mims, in
Thomasville, and Dr. Mims had agreed to give me a complete blood count on Monday, at ten in the morning.

I slept badly Saturday night. We had had a dove shoot
Saturday, and it had bothered me. When I was really sick—
when I was in close fear of Thanatos—I had no desire at all
to kill anything. "Neither will I again smite any more every
thing living, as I have done," God told Noah, and the phrase
kept coming back to me.

The quail shooting didn't bother me a bit. A quail is
really a miniature chicken, and there's surely nothing wrong
with killing a chicken to eat. Moreover, a quail almost always gives you a close, straight, going-away shot. Either you
kill it or you miss it—and if you do wound it, the dogs are
almost always sure to pick it up later, where you've marked
it down.

Dove shooting is different. Doves come swooping in
from all angles. They jog and swerve, which makes a hard
kill difficult. Above all, most of your shots are at extreme
range. Very often you know you have hit a dove, which
means it will almost surely die, but you don't pick it up. The
first three doves I hit came down in a field, and each in
succession got up again and flew off, wobbling in the air,
when the man who collects the birds tried to pick it up.

Dove are not little chickens, either. They are very beautiful birds, with their pink bellies and their blue-gray wings.
They are also symbols—Genesis, and Mount Ararat, and the

211

olive branch, and peace. Toward the end of the dove shoot, I was missing doves, sort of half on purpose; it is so easy to miss a dove that you don't have to try very hard. That Saturday night I had bad dreams—there was one terrible dream in which I shot at little Andrew, and he flopped about on the ground like a hit dove.

The next day, Sunday, I felt lousy, my stomach was queasy, I could only nibble at the delicious food, and in the evening I played bridge badly and lost, deserving to lose. The next morning, at ten, Tish drove me the few miles to Thomasville. It was a nice sunny day, and Dr. Mims had an office in a pleasant house surrounded by camelias in bloom. A nurse gave me a finger prick, and Dr. Mims told me to call about noon—he'd have the count by then.

Back in the Whitney guesthouse, I tried to work, but there was a small knot of fear in my belly. The blood is the mirror of the marrow, and if the counts were down, it could only mean that the bad cells were still gaining, maybe even, in John Glick's phrase, galloping. I kept looking at my pocket watch and called Dr. Mims precisely at noon.

"Why Mistuh Alsop," he said, "you have the blood of a perfectly normal man."

I felt like embracing him over the telephone.

Hemoglobin 15.1; white blood count 4,500, with 40 percent granulacytes; platelets more than doubled, to 151,000. I called John, and he said the counts were "marvelous." I think he's almost as relieved as I am. He warned me that an "eye count" could be pretty far off, as compared to the NIH machine count. But obviously the trend was in the right direction. Lovable Dr. Mims.

My stomach queasiness suddenly ended, my appetite came back with a rush, and I felt absolutely dandy. Such is the power of mind over matter.

Monday, January 31—

To NIH clinic for a blood test. Tish and I arrive at ten, and we chat for a while with John Glick—about George Wallace, and the Florida primary, and the South Bronx, subjects of recent journalistic expeditions. We talk briefly about the state of my health, which seems fine. John has tragic news: Tommy Thompson has just been readmitted to NIH, and the cancer has spread. It seems unlikely that he will leave the hospital alive.

I go to the finger-stick room and wait for the technicians to come in to take blood samples from the patients lined up on the chairs along the side of the room. It is a queer experience, this waiting in the finger-stick room. The room is hospital green, with the Christmas decorations still up. There are about ten of us sitting on the folding chairs, including a couple of mothers with small children on their laps. One quite pretty woman has an absolutely charming little girl of about three on her lap. The little girl probably has acute lymphoblastic leukemia. The technicians are late, and quiet conversations start.

To my left is a boy, about seventeen, and to his left is a girl, about a year older. They look like brother and sister. He has on a long light brown wig, and her wig is just the same color, and only a little longer. They both share the peculiar color of a leukemic who has had chemotherapy, a just barely discernible orangey tint to the skin and beneath the tint a pallor. The pallor, of course, comes from a low red blood count.

Boy: You in the hospital or the motel? (There is a motellike installation at NIH, for outpatients under treatment.)

213

Girl: I been in both. Now I'm in the hospital.

Boy: Which do you like better?

Girl: The hospital, I guess. The first day after my treatment, I feel so terrible, I'd rather be in the hospital.

Boy: I'd rather be in the motel. They don't bother you so much.

Pause.

Boy: You going home soon?

Girl: Maybe, if my counts are better.

Boy: Jeez, I hate waiting for the counts. He gets me in here at eight thirty, and then I have to wait around to get the finger stick, and then the waiting after that.

Girl: Yeah, I hate it too.

Another pause.

Boy: You wanta go out to the mall some night? (Mall? Maybe the Montgomery shopping mall?) Better than just sitting around.

Girl: Sure, I'd like that.

At this point the technician gestures, and the boy gets up to get his finger pricked.

Boy meets girl. But probably not for very long. They will both be lucky if they make twenty.

I get my finger prick and leave for the downtown office. John calls up at the office, as I am about to go to the White House for one of Henry Kissinger's lousy lunches. (The lunches sent up by the White House mess are almost inedible, but Henry is always interesting and amusing, though rarely very informative.) The platelets are down to 70,000, and the other counts are drifting downward. Maybe something's still in there, gnawing busily away. Or else, as John says, something happened, as a result of the allopurinol, which has permanently affected my marrow and my blood. If so, he says, it is something I can live with, maybe indefi-

214

nitely. My white blood count is low, John points out, but everybody else in town has had the flu, and I've not had so much as a sniffle.

Poor Tommy. Again, a wartime analogy occurs to me. John Glick at twenty-eight is in the supply corps; he might be hit by a bomb but only by damned bad luck. My six children are back in the States; they haven't even been drafted yet. Tish, at forty-four, with a history of arthritis and thrombosis, is in the light artillery. With my history, I'm in an infantry battalion at the front. Poor Tommy is the leader of the point platoon—and he's already been hit.

Wednesday, February 9

Tommy Thompson died at five last Monday at NIH, and his funeral was at twelve today, in the National Cathedral. Chip Bohlen, who is Tommy's twin—they were born within a few months of each other, and their careers marched in parallel—made a fine funeral oration, and he used just the right word about Tommy, the word "decent." Tommy was pre-eminently a decent man. Not that he was ever soft or silly; he was a tough and highly competitive man, as anyone who ever played bridge or poker with him can attest. But he also had a kind of instantly recognizable integrity, and that, combined with good sense and vast experience, gave him a special personal authority. People, including Presidents, listened to what he said and believed him.

When Charlie Bartlett and I interviewed Bobby Kennedy for our *Saturday Evening Post* piece on the Cuban missile crisis, I asked Kennedy which of the members of ExCom, the inner circle of Presidential advisers, had impressed him most during the crisis. He answered without hesitation, "Tommy."

215

Kennedy gave an example of Tommy's good sense. After the other side had "blinked" (from Dean Rusk's phrase, "We're eyeball to eyeball, and I think the other side just blinked"), Khrushchev ordered the ships sailing toward Cuba loaded with missile equipment to reverse course. The intelligence established that all the ships had done so—except one, which kept stolidly steaming toward Cuba.

The hawks, especially the military, chose to regard this as a deliberate provocation, a test of will, and proposed to bomb the Russian ship out of the water. Tommy quietly argued that it would be better to wait and see. Maybe that one ship hadn't got the message; maybe the wireless operator had been drunk or asleep. The President agreed. In a couple of hours the ship awoke with a start, as it were, and hastily reversed course.

I went to see Jane Thompson yesterday. Tommy, she said, died without pain—rare in cancer of the pancreas—and in his lucid moments he was cheerful and even funny. He suddenly asked her, "Have you ever played millstone bridge?" and then went on to define millstone bridge as the kind of bridge in which your partner is a millstone round your neck.

She recalled one of Tommy's favorite Khrushchev stories. During the U-2 blowup at the Paris summit in 1960, Khrushchev came up to Tommy and stepped hard on his instep and said, "Excuse me," in Russian.

"Why did you do that?" asked Tommy.

"Because in Russia when we do something like that, we apologize," said Khrushchev. "Why don't you apologize for the U-2?"

Tommy also loved the story about Jane and the dance at the Kremlin. During his first tour as Ambassador, as the thaw began, he and Jane were asked to a party at the Kremlin, complete with dancing—something quite unknown in the Stalin era. A middle-level Soviet official approached Jane, whose Junoesque figure was much admired by the Russians, and asked her to dance.

"Do you waltz?" asked Jane.

"Naw," said the Russian. "I do not waltz. Is too old-fashioned. I fox. Sometimes I fox quick, sometimes I fox slow. All depends on what the lady likes."

I can hear Tommy, in my mind's ear, laughing his small heh-heh-heh giggle at this story.* He won't laugh again, poor fellow. His death has moved me more than most, not only because I liked and admired him but because we were both told we had an inoperable cancer at almost the same time last summer. He died on Monday, and I played three sets of indoor tennis on Tuesday. But his death serves as a reminder, an intimation of mortality.

\|\|\|\|\|\|\|\|\|\|\|\|\|\|\|\|\|\|\|\|\|\|\|\|\|\|\|\|\|\|\|\|\|\|\|\|\|\|\|\|\|\|\|\|\|\|\|\|\|\|\|\|\|\|\|\|\|\|\|\|\|\|\|\|\|

Robert Burns (I thought it was Alexander Pope before I looked it up in Bartlett's) wrote of "man's inhumanity to man." Hardly anybody writes about nature's cruelty to man. But nature's cruelty is, at its most horrible, more horrible than man's.

Leukemics are lucky in some ways. A terminal leukemic is not a pretty sight, but with a wig and a bit of effort he or she still looks more or less human. Wandering about the NIH clinical center, in the corridors or in the elevator, one

---

* Jane Thompson tells me I have the story all wrong. But I like it as it is.

comes occasionally on a human monster, on a living nightmare, on a face or body hideously deformed.

I remember especially a young man—he must have been under twenty—who had a cancer which had turned his skin into a strange, coppery leather. He must have had other forms of cancer too; he talked in a kind of monotone shriek, suggesting some damage to the larynx, and his legs and arms twitched like a marionette's. He was seated in a waiting room when I saw him, and then he started to get up, using a sort of two-handled cane on little wheels. He was as awkward as a newborn colt trying to rise to its feet, and intolerably painful to watch. What had this young man done, I asked myself, to deserve this?

Leukemics are lucky in another way too. Most leukemics die of fungal or bacterial infection, pneumonia being a much-used exit, although there are also occasional deaths by hemorrhage when platelet rejection has occurred. These are relatively painless ways of dying. Some cancers impose on their victims unimaginable suffering before they are allowed to die. This suffering is, after all, the work of dear old Mother Nature.

There have always been "nature-fakers," in Theodore Roosevelt's phrase, but never more so than now. The "mother earth" myth has led a lot of people, young people especially, to suppose that Mother Nature is wonderfully benign. In fact, nature is cruel, inherently and unchangeably cruel.

Even the vegetable world is engaged always in a savage and ruthless competition for survival, as anyone who has left a garden untended for a few weeks can attest. As for the animal world, from the ocean or the feed lot up to the dinner table, it operates on the principle that stronger or cleverer animals have the right and duty to eat smaller or stupider animals. Human beings, fortunately, are less stupid than other animals, which makes it possible for us to munch daily on the flesh and blood of some peace-loving Hereford or Black Angus, if we have the money, or, if we have less, on the hindquarters of an amiable pig or the leg of a inoffensive chicken.

Nature can be more cruel than man, but man's inhumanity to man is an abiding reality of all history. The idealistic young who refuse to recognize this reality are courting a painful disillusionment.

I remember a talk with a very tall, very handsome young man in a coffeehouse—a center of the antiwar underground—near Fort Dix, in New Jersey, in 1969, at the height of the Vietnam war. The young man was just out of law school, and he had joined an antiwar commune and intended to devote all his time to defending enlisted men who got into trouble with the military for antiwar activities.

He seemed to me a most impressive young man. He held forth eloquently on the iniquities of the capitalist-imperialist system, and although this was old stuff mostly, familiar since freshman year at Yale, he was articulate and impressively sincere.

What system, I asked, should be substituted? Perhaps some form of Marxism? Ownership by the state of the means of production and distribution? No, he said, none of that; he had taken a trip to Russia and Eastern Europe, and he saw that people were even less free there than in America.

"What we want," he said, "is a society in which there is no government at all, and people live together in accord with nature and love each other." Then he looked at me searchingly, with large, liquid brown eyes. "I can see in your eyes you don't believe in that."

"No, I don't," I said, and did not try to explain why.

I wonder what's happened to that young man. Maybe a striving junior partner in his law firm, stepping on the faces of other junior partners in order to become a senior partner? Or maybe, "in accord with nature," he is writhing with bone cancer? Life will be cruel to him in the end, in any case. "Golden lads and girls all must, as chimney-sweepers, come to dust."

All this suggests why I find it difficult to believe in a "just and merciful God." How just? In what way merciful?

If there is a God, he must be a savage and unpredictable deity, ruling more by fear than by love. A line from Fourth Form Latin pops into the mind: *Primum in orbe deos fecit timor*—"Fear first made gods in the world." The fear is there, buried deep in the psyche, below the layer of cool reason and an open-minded agnosticism. One wants to put a chip on the double zero, just in case. Please God, please Mother, please Father, please Aggie.

Perhaps it is just that Tommy Thompson's death has depressed me.

Tuesday, February 15—

Noon. Into the clinic today for blood and marrow tests. Feeling fine, filled with a secret hope that the percentage of bad cells would be nicely down. The marrow was relatively painless and quick and the technician said there were plenty of spicules. Tish and I didn't want to wait with the Nos Morituri Brigade, so John promised to call us at home with the results, at about noon.

He just called. I could tell from his voice that the results were not good. It seems that the technician was wrong; there were no spicules, so I have to go back at one thirty for another marrow test. This is the first time this has happened.

Also, the platelets are badly down, to 43,000.

John obviously suspects that the bad cells are increasing, killing or crowding out the megakaryocytes, the cells that produce platelets. But if so, what does it mean, and what will happen to me? As usual, he doesn't know the answer to either question. Nobody knows.

This damnable experience is more and more like the old serial movie, *The Perils of Pauline,* that brother John and I used to see at the weekly movie shows at the Avon town hall. I wish I didn't know so much. If John Glick told me nothing, I'd happily play tennis this afternoon, happily go off shooting at Mac Herter's next week. Instead, there is again that consciousness of the Damocletian sword, that small pea of fear at the back of the mind.

Four p.m. John just called. The Damocletian sword has become a bit heavier, the pea a bit bigger.

I was "remarrowed"—hateful verb—at one thirty, and I also had a biopsy, a section of bone and flesh. Both painful—apparently, the more painful, the more successful.

John said that the cells were definitely up—17 percent bad cells by one count, 16 percent by another. There were also fewer megakaryocytes, and less "granulocytic activity" in the marrow.

John had just had a long talk with Dr. Henderson and the other doctors. All agreed that there should be no chemotherapy now. But there is, as usual, no agreement on what is wrong with me. John says, "Nothing fits." Dr. Henderson, asked what he would guess if he had to, replied that he would have to guess that I had some form of wholly idiosyncratic leukemia—"Alsop's leukemia," in John's phrase.

What to do? For the present, nothing. Learn to live with it. If the platelets go down to the danger point, I'll have platelet transfusions. If the percentage of bad cells continues to climb, they may try steroids or a mild form of outpatient chemotherapy.

I felt fine this morning. Now I feel lousy. Did John have to tell me? The question had obviously occurred to him.

"If this were another kind of hospital, and you were another kind of patient, I'd have told you the counts were stable. But it's the policy here to tell the patient the truth. And you'd never have stood for a bland answer anyway. You have too inquiring a mind."

Well, maybe. But I'm not so sure. A frightened man welcomes a certain blandness. I think I would be capable of a remarkable degree of self-deception, if only John would let me deceive myself.

February 17—

I called Dr. Djerassi, and we had a long talk. He had been in Paris and spent two days with Dr. Mathé, the genius of the Pasteur Institute who has invented a technique for immunizing patients with threatened leukemia. They had discussed my case, and they agreed that some sort of self-immunizing process was probably at work. At any rate, the case didn't call for immunotherapy, except as a last resort. As for the Mathé technique, it was much more effective against acute lymphoblastic leukemia, or ALL, than against AML, and I couldn't possibly have ALL.

I told Dr. Djerassi what John had told me—that there was no evidence of auto-immunity in my blood tests. Djerassi rather brushed this aside. Auto-immunity was often impossible to detect. If he had to guess, he said, he would guess that I did not have leukemia, that the abnormal cells were mimic cells rather than true malignant cells, and that I represented "some sort of complicated auto-immune situation." This is a more encouraging guess than Dr. Henderson's.

Cheeha Combahee Plantation, S.C.
February 20—

Tracy Barnes is dead. He went into his house in Rhode Island and collapsed in the hallway like a felled ox with a massive heart attack. Like a felled ox—the cliché fits Tracy. I saw him a few days ago, at Tommy Thompson's funeral, and he looked, as he always looked, strong as an ox. But he'd had a couple of strokes, and the heart attack was not unexpected.

Shakespeare doesn't have to be rewritten for Tracy Barnes. I'm sure he never tasted of death but once, despite those previous strokes. He was a couple of forms ahead of me at Groton, but I only got to know him well in wartime London, when he was an OSS paratrooper. He jumped behind the lines, not once but twice. The rest of us considered one jump into occupied territory as much as could reasonably be expected of us.

Tracy stayed on with the intelligence apparat after the war, and he was number two to Dick Bissell (another Grotonian and old friend) when Bissell was in charge of the Bay of Pigs operation. They had both made brilliant records before the Bay of Pigs. Bissell, for example, was primarily responsible for the aerial surveillance of the Soviet Union —first by U-2, then by satellite—that now chiefly ensures the relative stability of the nuclear equation. After the Bay of Pigs, President Kennedy told Allen Dulles and Dick Bissell, "Under the British system, I would have to go. Under our system, I'm afraid it has to be you."

Bissell and Dulles went. Tracy Barnes stayed on in CIA for some years—unwisely, since the Bay of Pigs had put its mark on him—and then went to work for Yale. He was not only very brave, he was great fun to be with. He was just sixty when he died. Maybe sixty is a good age to die at.

223

Most of us here at Cheeha Combahee were good friends of Tracy and would have gone to the funeral in Rhode Island. But Janet Barnes, bless her, insisted stubbornly that she wanted no one but family, and thus our South Carolina quail-shooting week was saved.

Tish and I have been coming here for a week in the winter for fifteen years now, thanks to Mac Herter—more formally, Mrs. Christian A. Herter. Chris Herter, Secretary of State in the last Eisenhower years, died in 1966. Andrew Alsop's middle name is Christian, in his memory.

This place is very different from Greenwood, the Jock Whitney place. Greenwood is a handsome, pillared, ante-bellum mansion, bought by a Whitney shortly after the Civil War. It has gardens of startling beauty, and every guest has a large bedroom filled with priceless prints and a bathroom all to himself. The food is justly famous, and at dinner the wine is apt to be a Lafitte '61 or a Margaux '49 or the like.

The house at Cheeha Combahee is a shooting lodge, built in 1929. It is a handsome but unpretentious one-story house with two wings. There are six double bedrooms in one wing, and a dining room, kitchen, and living room in the other. The whole place is heated entirely by wood fires; I am writing this before a cheerful fire in bedroom number 6. There is one bathroom for the ladies, and one for the men, each with a two-holer. In 1959, when Tom Gates was a fellow guest, I went into the bathroom after breakfast and found both places already occupied by the Secretary of State and the Secretary of Defense. I could not help but be impressed.

The house is surrounded by a bright green expanse of rye grass, with camellia bushes and live oaks bearded with Spanish moss. The food is delicious but simple—quail cooked outdoors in bacon fat for lunch, local shad or beef or ham for dinner. Chris Herter used to cook the luncheon quail. I have a vivid mental image of him fanning the frying pan with his hat, to put out the fire when the bacon fat flared up. The wine, until some finicky guests rebelled, was Virginia Dare.

Both places are, in a sense, courtesy of old John D. Rockefeller. Both Jock Whitney and Mac Herter had forebears sensible enough to go into partnership with the ruthless old genius. Both places afford a wonderfully pleasurable week-long house party to those lucky enough to be asked as guests, with lots of talk, lots of bridge, and lots of quail shooting.

Father used to be asked to various quail-shooting plantations every winter. My brother John and his wife Gussie are here this week, and they make regular pilgrimages to a couple of other quail-shooting plantations. In short, we Alsops are almost professional quail-shooting guests.

I vaguely remember a scene from a nineteenth-century English novel (I think it was a novel. Trollope, perhaps? Or was it a joke in *Punch*? Or did I make it up?) in which the Duke and his Duchess are discussing the guest list for the grouse shooting. The Duke proposes Mr. So-and-so. The Duchess objects: "But isn't he a bit of a cad?" The Duke replies: "Of course he's a cad, but he's a good shot and he plays a decent game of whist." I tell John that we are asked South every year for much the same reasons.

John is, by common consent, the most entertaining of the three Alsop brothers. He may also be the best writer— he was editor-in-chief of the *Grotonian*, whereas Joe and I were mere associate editors. Gussie can be funnier than John, especially when she is describing why it's necessary to hit John occasionally with a blunt object to keep him in his place. They are both very good value on a week-long house party like this one, except in one way. The one way is the way John shoots quail.

John is a very good shot, and a very fast shot. We are

225

often paired, and it drives me crazy. A bird gets up, and there is a BANG-BANG. The second *bang* is always mine, and the bird is almost always already dead by the time I pull the trigger. This exacerbates my sense of sibling rivalry. The Alsop brothers are fond of each other, but there is plenty of sibling rivalry between us.

Nonshooting friends of mine are mystified by my passion for shooting at quail. It is hard to explain. Chip Bohlen says that Russia is like the act of love—it cannot be explained, it can only be experienced. That is true of quail-shooting too.

Our shooting party yesterday consisted of eight people, on eight horses, plus a pickup truck with six dogs. We brought home nine quail. A quail is a small bird, not much bigger than a robin. The hunter-hunted ratio in terms of weight must be more than 100,000 to 1. Granted that the little birds make delicious eating, is that any way for sensible grown-up people to spend hours at a time?

You sit on an old horse, as it plods through fields and through woods. Out front the dogs quarter back and forth, sniffing for quail, covering acre after acre like vacuum cleaners. The sun filters at a slanted angle through the live oaks and turns the sedge grass a golden brown. The horse plods on, and you sit on his back, and you find yourself thinking in a way you don't often have time to think—lazily, at random, for pleasure. You remember a bit of poetry or a snatch of song, you remember a girl you once liked very much and had almost forgotten, or you remember something that happened long ago that amused or interested you.

I inherited from Father a good Winchester double-barreled twelve gauge—not a great gun like a Purdy but a good, reliable, serviceable big gun. Pa's initials, JWA, are embossed on a little gold plaque on the stock. The gun is

226

carried in a holster beside the saddle and yesterday, glancing down at the gun, I saw Pa's initials winking in the sun and began to think about Pa.

The gun is between forty and fifty years old, and in my mind's eye I could see Pa, two inches taller than I, and heavier, with a big nose like mine, plodding along on some now-long-dead horse, waiting for the dogs to point all those long years ago. Pa was about to go on a quail hunt when he died at seventy-seven, here in South Carolina, in 1952. He is dead, but there is still a lot of Pa alive in me, I thought. I have Pa's nose and forehead and his legs, with big feet, round calves, and thin shanks.

When I die, I thought, there will be a lot of me still alive in my six children—probably more of me in Joe and Elizabeth than in the others, and least in Ian, or maybe Andrew, both of whom are very visibly Tish's children. There are other ways in which Pa is still alive in me. For example, he infected me and John with the passion for shooting and fishing (it never took with Joe). Too bad, I thought, that I have never been able to infect my children. They say they are against killing things, and in a way perhaps they're right.

I was thinking this yesterday when the huntsman's hand went up, and somebody yelled "Point!" A dog was standing rigid, its tail straight out, its belly close to the ground, the other dog loyally backing him a few yards away. It was my turn to shoot, and I slid off the horse, pulled my gun out of the holster, and put two shells into the chambers.

The first dog began to creep forward, on tiptoe. "Careful," said Bob MacMillan, the huntsman, urgently. "Careful, Rebel." Paul Nitze was shooting with me this time—fortunately not brother John—and we walked up quickly be-

227

hind the dogs, our guns ready. Although I had done this a thousand times and more, my heart was beating a little fast, as always.

Nothing happened. The dogs crept forward again, stealthily. Still nothing happened. "Maybe a false point," I said, and just as I said the word "point," the covey rose, with that familiar, always surprising whir of feathers, and I had my gun without thinking at my shoulder, with the safety off. I missed the first shot, disgracefully, but killed the bird with the second shot. Paul Nitze killed two birds. Three birds with four shots is good shooting. "Good work," said Bob MacMillan, who is sparing of compliments.

Perhaps the children are right about not wanting to kill things, but they miss something curiously and inexplicably exciting and pleasurable.

Back on the horse, I began to think again, and I found myself grinning a little to myself. The Duke and Duchess and the cad had reminded me of something that had happened, back in the early fifties, to me.

I was in London, on a reporting trip for Joe's and my column. I had an introduction to Lord Salisbury and interviewed him—he was a powerful figure in those days—and he asked me for the weekend to his country seat, Hatfield House. On a Friday afternoon, I drew up before the ancient pile, built by Salisbury's ancestor, Sir Robert Cecil, first minister to Queen Elizabeth and James I.

I paid off the taxi and timidly rang a doorbell. To my surprise, Lady Salisbury, a gray-haired lady with a strong ancestral face, answered the bell. With her was an enormous hound, which looked at me in a markedly unfriendly fashion and growled.

When I was a little boy, and Pa and I were walking along a road near our Connecticut farm, a big dog leapt off the porch of a house and ran straight at me, growling and barking. Pa told me to pay no attention, that a dog would never bite unless he smelt "the acrid smell of fear." Ever since then, when a dog growls at me, I exude the acrid smell of fear in great quantities. The enormous hound seemed to be smelling it.

Lady Salisbury may have smelled it too. At any rate, she saw that I was nervous. "Don't worry," she said. "Bobo never bites a gentleman, only tradesmen or the lower classes."

At this point, Bobo lunged forward and planted his teeth in my right calf. It was an embarrassing moment for Lady Salisbury, and more so for me.

Wednesday, March 1—

This morning I made a deal with John Glick. He agreed to it with surprising ease.

I had a wonderful time at Cheeha Combahee plantation, until the day before we came home. Mac Herter was in fine form; she seems completely recovered from her lung cancer operation. There was good company—John and Gussie, the Russell Trains, the Paul Nitzes, toward the end of the week, the young Chris Herters and Bill and Jill Ruckelshaus. There was good talk, good shooting, and good eating. But on Friday, the last full day, I began to feel lousy.

Nothing specific, just a kind of queasiness, a malaise. Why? Because I knew that I would have a blood test on Monday and that, if the results were not good, John Glick would do a marrow test to find out what was going on? Or did I have some sort of bug?

When I went in for the test on Monday, I told John I had been feeling low, and he obviously suspected my low

229

feelings were psychosomatic in origin. He recalled the case of a patient who came in for a test with a container of vomit. The patient thought the vomit should be analyzed, to determine what was wrong with him, but all that was wrong with him was that he was terrified of what the test might show. John took some blood and called at the office that afternoon to say that there had been a clot in the blood. The clot threw off the results of the test, so would I please come in again for a finger stick?

I had the finger stick Tuesday morning, with the rest of the Nos Morituri Brigade, and John called with the results at about eleven. Not good. Not at all good. The hemoglobin is holding up, but the platelets and the granulocytes are both sharply down.

Something is obviously going on, and whatever it is, it's not good. John theorized that whatever is wrong with me may be cyclic. Perhaps the allopurinol was not the key factor; perhaps in October I just hit the up cycle. Now I am in a down cycle. In any case, John said, there is nothing to do but wait and see. Even if the bad cells are again up, to around 25 percent, say (which he obviously suspects), we'll still wait and see. He asked me to come in for another blood test on Friday and, unless there's a sharp improvement, a marrow on Monday.

I had a lunch date with Kay Graham at the Sans Souci. I called her and told her I had some lousy news about my blood, and that I couldn't face all those genial friends at Sans Souci. So she asked me to lunch at her house, and we talked, and after lunch I felt much more cheerful, and I made a decision.

John had told me that, bar some catastrophic fulmination, nothing would be done anyway. So why was it necessary to face these endless prickings and probings, the Nos Morituri Brigade, and, perhaps worst of all, the waiting for the results of the tests? I talked it over with Tish that evening and decided to ask John the next day for a one-month vacation from all tests of any sort. I called him from the office this morning; rather to my surprise, he agreed without a murmur and added that it might be a very good idea. I am to call him if I have a temperature or bleeding or anything else goes seriously wrong. Otherwise, no prickings and probings until April.

I feel like a boy let out of school. No more lessons, no more books, no more teacher's dirty looks. No more blood tests, no more marrows, no more biopsies—at least for a month. I hadn't realized how all those prickings and probings had been getting me down, almost more than the bad results of the tests.

Tuesday, March 21—

Here we go again. Back to square one.

John Glick and I had agreed on a vacation from the green walls and the dying people of the NIH clinic for a month—till April 3. The vacation ended early today.

I had a toothache, very much like the toothaches I had last spring before I was diagnosed as a leukemic. The toothache started on Sunday, and it got worse on Monday. I had it in mind to go to Dr. Baxter and get it fixed and say nothing to John Glick, but Tish insisted on calling John—she was right, of course, for low platelets involve the danger of hemorrhaging. John said I had to have a blood count. I hated the idea, because I didn't want to go back to the damnable clinic, and I didn't want to worry about my damnable blood count, and also I knew, somehow, that the count would be bad. Although I've been wholly operational, I've been feeling more like August than November.

Tish drove me to NIH for the ten-thirty finger stick.

231

There was a pathetic girl in her teens, very white, with bad skin, who looked as though she hadn't too long to go, and another cheerful woman with a ravaged complexion who looked very sick indeed. Waiting for the finger stick, we chatted with John briefly—he's just back from Nassau and looks well, or at least less pallid than usual.

John said he'd thought in Nassau about what I'd said when I asked for the vacation from NIH—how terribly tired I'd become of my own blood and marrow counts, how I wanted never again to hear words like platelets and granulocytes. Perhaps, John said, I'd rather not have my counts any more; he would treat me if I needed treatment, but if not, I could forget about the counts. I told him I'd been thinking along the same lines. The only trouble was that I wanted to hear any good news, and if he didn't tell me good news, I'd assume, by a simple process of elimination, that the news was bad—and I might imagine it was even worse than it really was.

I said I'd think it over, and he said he'd call Tish at home with the counts. I went to the office and called her after twelve, when she hadn't called me. I had a sense of foreboding, and it grew when she told me John hadn't called —obviously, the counts had surprised him, and he'd asked for a recount. Knowing John, I knew that if the surprise had been a pleasant one, he'd have called right away.

I called Tish again at about one. She said that John had said the results didn't call for treatment, at least not yet.

"So what were the counts?" I asked.

"Do you really want to know?" she said.

"Yes," I said.

Hemoglobin down to 14.1—not too bad. Platelets at 25,000 just above the danger zone of 20,000. Granulocyte count just at the danger point of 500.

Not at all good. John says with this kind of count I

ought to have another blood count next week, whether I have a marrow test or not. Except for the hemoglobin, I'm back to the lousy counts of August. John told Tish that if the marrow count goes to 50 percent or more abnormal cells—which I suspect he now suspects it will—he will give me chemotherapy. But it will not be the horror of the laminar flow room; it will be a relatively mild chemotherapy, taken by mouth as well as intravenously, on an outpatient basis, rather than the "aggressive protocol" for AML. He's sure I don't have AML. He still doesn't know what I do have.

I had two martinis at lunch, on the grounds that I deserved them. I played tennis, and pretty well, and we had a pleasant evening with Tom and Joan Braden. But the pea is back. I remember a game we used to play in Avon as children. An object would be held over a child's head, and the other children would intone, "Heavy, heavy, what hangs over?" If the child guessed wrong, he was It, and all the other children would run away from him.

There is something grim about the phrase "Heavy, heavy, what hangs over?" In the last few days, it has kept popping back into my mind.

Tuesday, April 4—

This is Wisconsin primary day, and I've spent a good deal of time wondering about the outcome of the primary, and also wondering about whether I shall die soon, mostly the former.

This was the day agreed on with John Glick a month ago for my next blood and marrow tests. I was prepared for bad news anyway before I went for my marrow test at three this afternoon. I was the more prepared, because of what happened this morning.

I got up feeling pretty spry, went to the bathroom,

233

blew my large nose, and a nosebleed started. Nothing to worry about, I said to myself; lots of people have nosebleeds. But I knew there was something to worry about when the nosebleed refused to stop. I went back to bed, and Tish brought up some ice in a plastic bag. I lay with my nose freezing for about a half an hour and then went to the bathroom to shave and shower. In the shower, I blew my nose gently and the nosebleed started again. I went back to bed and lay there freezing my nose until eleven. Then I got up, and this time the clot held. But I also knew by this time what the nosebleed meant—low platelets.

I'd meant to go to the office, to do some preliminary telephoning for a Wisconsin piece, but with the marrow coming up at three, and my damnable nose still feeling as though it were about to start bleeding again, I called Amanda and told her I'd skip it. I read the papers more thoroughly than usual. Reread a piece I'd written over the weekend at Needwood and realized it was no good, except for one phrase ("the clothespin vote," for Democrats who will vote for Nixon with vast reluctance). Tried to write a better piece, and failed, and worried about the tests that afternoon.

I told John Glick that I wanted to know only two things: if there had been a real turn for the better, or if there had been such a turn for the worse that some action had to be taken—a transfusion, for example, or chemotherapy of some sort. John readily agreed. I think his lengthening experience as an oncologist is beginning to give him doubts about whether it is really a good idea to tell a cancer patient everything.

The marrow test wasn't too bad. There was a nice black nurse who patted me when my legs twitched, and John got spicules the first time in. Then he drew some blood and asked us to stay while he had a quick look at the marrow and the blood. After less than half an hour, he came into the operating room where Tish and I were waiting.

"I'm not going to give you the counts, as we agreed," he said, "but there's a decision that has to be made, and I want some advice, so I'll call you later at home, maybe in a couple of hours."

"The decision is whether to give me a platelet transfusion, isn't it, John?" I asked.

"Yes," he said.

"Is the platelet count under twenty thousand?" I asked.

"You really want to know?" he asked.

I nodded.

"Yes, it's under twenty thousand. But the news isn't all bad. Your granulocytes are actually up a bit, and your hemoglobin's normal." He confessed himself mystified all over again. "I was developing a pretty firm theory, but I can't account for this—your platelets way down and your hemoglobin steady and your granulocyte count actually up. It just doesn't fit."

John called later to say that there would be no transfusion and no chemotherapy, at least for the present. He is betting on the proposition that the disease is cyclic and that, as in September, the counts will suddenly improve. I hope —Please God, please Mother, please Father, please Aggie— he is right.

April 14—

Yesterday I played tennis, and on the way to dinner and bridge with the Johnnie Walkers, I told Tish I was

235

feeling pretty pooped and I was afraid my hemoglobin was down.

"Yes," she said, "John Glick called and said to tell you you could play tennis if you felt up to it, but not to try too hard."

I had had a blood test the day before, but, as agreed, John had not called me with the counts.

"Oh," I said. "You talked to John. Did he give you the counts?"

"Yes."

"What were they?"

"Do you really want to know?"

I hesitated briefly. "Yes," I said.

"Hemoglobin a bit above twelve, not too bad. Platelets eighteen thousand. WBC twenty-seven hundred."

"What percentage granulocytes?"

"Ten percent."

"Only two seventy. Jesus."

We drove in silence the rest of the way to the Walkers and lost every rubber.

Today I called John, and we talked at some length on the telephone. What it all amounted to was that I'm right back where I started from. John clearly expects the hemoglobin count to follow the other counts down into the cellar. That's what I dread most—or, to be honest, second most. (What I dread most is getting very sick and dying.) You feel so lousy when your hemoglobin is low. And how am I to cover a Presidential campaign if I can barely drag myself around?

It is full spring now, the lovely Washington April. But T. S. Eliot was right. April is the cruelest month.

Most of my friends wrote me a letter when I first got sick and thereafter, quite naturally, left it at that. But there were a couple of exceptions.

Tom Braden, the lance corporal in the King's Royal Rifle Corps who met me outside the officers' mess in Winchester and reported to Ted Ellsworth that I was a *real* horse's ass, is now, after a variegated career, a fellow Washington columnist. He is, I suppose, my best friend, and Tish and I see a lot of him and his famously charming wife, Joan. Joan is my second most assiduous correspondent. She wrote me every day when I was in the hospital, and when she is away—she and Tom are restless travelers—she always writes, which cheers me up.

But my most assiduous correspondent was—and still is, as I write—an interesting fellow called Peter B. Young. Peter B. Young was the first to suggest that I keep a journal. "I can see the dust cover now," he wrote. "The BIG LUKE DIARY, My Nineteen-Month Battle with Leukemia, by Stewart Alsop." Later, he wrote me a long series of letters describing in detail his sufferings from a peculiarly revolting disease, "athlete's ass." In a note to Amanda Zimmerman he explained his motives:

"Dear Amanda: Haven't you heard of shock therapy? My strategy was to discuss in excruciating, disgusting detail *my* medical problem. It's not that I'm vulgar and crude by nature (though I am); it was planning, baby, planning."

Pete Young has been more useful to me journalistically than a whole covey of State Department or Pentagon leaks handing out Top Secret papers by the bushel basket. I met him in an odd way. Shortly after the Watts riot in Los Angeles in 1965, I went out to Watts to talk to people and try to understand why the riot had happened. With Andrew Jaffe, who had done a brilliant job covering the Watts

237

riots for the AP (and who is now with *Newsweek*) as my guide, I spent a long day of walking and talking in Watts. For the first time, I sensed the depth of the bitterness of many blacks, especially the young, a bitterness toward all white people that seemed ineradicable, automatic, a learned response. As I wrote for my column in the *Saturday Evening Post*, "in Watts, for the first time, it began to seem to me that the racial problem in this country is wholly insoluble—that it is like some incurable disease, with which both whites and Negroes must learn to live in pain, all the days of our lives."

After the *Post* published my column, I got a telegram: SO NOW YOU'VE SEEN THE BLACK GHETTO. COME TO GREENE COUNTY NORTH CAROLINA KNOWN AS KU KLUX KLAN CAPITAL USA AND SEE THE WHITE GHETTO. SIGNED PETER B. YOUNG.

My curiosity was aroused. I telephoned Peter B. Young, who turned out to be a television newsman in Raleigh, North Carolina. He claimed to know the Ku Klux Klan better than any other non-Klansman. I owed it to myself and my readers, he said, to understand and describe the other side of the Watts coin—"the anguish and despair of the white ghetto."

My native caution was also aroused, and I checked with a couple of North Carolina newspaper friends. Pete Young, I was told, was "hipped on the Klan" and "clever but somewhat eccentric." But at least, both agreed, Young was not dangerous. Sometimes I've wondered if they were right. Because of Peter B. Young, I have found myself in some rather sticky situations.

I decided to accept Young's invitation to visit the Klan. I also decided to invite Ted Ellsworth along. After the war, Ted returned to the insurance business, in Dubuque, Iowa, but he is always ready to embark on an adventure. Inviting Ellsworth turned out to be a brilliant idea. The Ku

Kluxers found me a cold Northern fish, but they immediately took to Ellsworth; they even offered him the Grand Dragonship of Iowa. They talked to him as they would never have talked to me.

Ellsworth came to Washington, and we flew together to Raleigh. At the airport we met Peter B. Young and Raymond Cranford, Exalted Cyclops of the Greene County Ku Klux Klan. They were an odd pair. Peter B. Young is a grandson of Brigham Young. (He must have a great many cousins, since the Mormon leader had seventeen wives and forty-seven children.) Pete may have inherited the spiritual peculiarities of his grandfather, but he does not look a bit like a Mormon prophet. He is short, with close-cropped hair, and even back in 1965, when he was thirty-three, he was contending with a small pot. He is also, as we soon discovered on that trip, an entertaining fellow, with an original mind and a unique talent.

The Exalted Cyclops, Raymond Cranford, also wore his hair cropped short, but in every other way he was as different from Pete Young as it is possible to be. He was a great hulking brute of a man, with a slit of a mouth, a bullet head, and light, expressionless eyes. The four of us sat down for lunch at the Raleigh airport and were immediately treated to the conversational style of the Exalted Cyclops.

"A white nigger, that's worse than a nigger. A white nigger's a man's got a white skin, and a heart that's pumpin' nigger blood through his veins. If it comes to a fight, the white nigger's gonna get killed before the nigger. . . . We believe a white man's got his civil rights too. I'll lay down my life for those rights, if I have to. These nigger civil rights, they're gonna end in the white man's bedroom. . . . When the Communists take over, they're gonna kill me quick. Well, you only got one time to die. . . ."

239

For four days, almost literally *ad nauseam,* we endured that kind of conversation. We spent those four days rushing about in cars, inspecting the Klaverns—sad little Klan meeting halls built of cinder block—eating heavily fried food, and enduring the nigger talk. All the Klansmen kept guns in their cars and on their persons. It was clear that to these people a gun is a phallic symbol, a proof of manhood.

In the end, it seemed to me that the Klansmen were more pathetic than evil. These farmers and gas station attendants and small shopkeepers felt as excluded from the "white power structure" as the young blacks of Watts. Their guns and their Klaverns and their rituals and their near-regulation service uniforms were pathetic substitutes for a grim or tedious reality. The trouble is, of course, that the guns of the Klan, like the guns in the black ghetto, are not play guns. They are real, and they are loaded.

That visit to the Klan, on the heels of the visit to Watts, gave me a foreboding sense of the fragility of American society, of the threat of violence that lies always close below the surface. So have many of the other expeditions which I have since undertaken with Peter B. Young.

I used to resist, after that visit to the Klan, when Pete would call up and say, "Sergeant Young, here, reporting for duty. Colonel, sir, we are mounting another expedition."

I resist no longer. Now I say, "Okay, Pete, where are we going this time?"

Pete has led me on expeditions to interview the black militant leaders in Harlem; to an army coffeehouse run by radical dissidents at the height of the Vietnam war; to Paul Krassner, David Dellinger, and other radical bellwethers in the heyday of the New Left; to Toronto to interview the draft dodgers and deserters there; to a kind of heroin speakeasy close to Central Park; to the South Bronx, to examine the process that is causing the black slums to be physically destroyed; to the Tombs; twice to Newark, for the smell of a city in full decay; and to other places I would never have visited on my own initiative.

Every one of these expeditions has paid off, not only in good copy but in my own understanding of the angry and alienated subcultures that underlie the affluent surface of American life. I have sometimes wondered what is in it for Pete, other than a chance to stay for free at a Holiday Inn. (He has a strange passion for Holiday Inns, and whenever we mount an expedition he always makes reservations at one.) Perhaps, having a unique talent, he likes to exercise it, using me as a sort of medium.

One of my expeditions with Pete Young had a rather embarrassing postscript. I had gone to New York with Pete to interview, among others, David Dellinger, the elder statesman of the New Left. After a few minutes of conversation, we suddenly recognized each other, through the fleshy incrustations of the years, as Yale classmates. I conceived a certain reluctant respect for Dave, for his willingness to go to jail (he has spent several years in jail) for ideas with which I totally disagree. In 1968, he and several other New Leftists were summoned to Washington to testify before the House Un-American Activities Committee. I asked David Dellinger to lunch at a fashionable French restaurant frequented by the Washington establishment and suggested that he might like to have a friend or two along.

Dellinger showed up half an hour late. He was not alone. Abbie Hoffman was with him, with a long white feather in his mop of hair. Jerry Rubin appeared naked to the waist, with a toy M-16. Paul Krassner, editor of *The Realist*, showed up in some outlandish costume, and they

241

were accompanied by a big silent black and three girls dressed as witches. I had thought that the liberated pot generation did not drink, but this turned out to be an illusion (an expensive one for *Newsweek*), and the table was soon loudly merry. Attempting to justify my expense account, I tried to interview Abbie Hoffman.

"Mr. Hoffman, I wish you would explain to me the goals of your movement."

At this point our table fell silent for the first time, and since the other tables had long since been reduced to bemused silence, the whole restaurant was still.

"ABOLISH PAY TOILETS, MAN!" shouted Hoffman at the top of his voice, while all heads turned in our direction. "That's the goal of the revolution—eternal life and free toilets!"

To an extraordinary extent, the New Left of that period —the height of the Vietnam war—was a jape or put-on. It was never the serious revolutionary movement many middle-class sobersides took it to be. And yet, while it lasted, the New Left undoubtedly changed the course of American history. Before the Chicago convention, Jerry Rubin was asked what he planned to do in Chicago. "Like, maybe, destroy the Democratic Party," he replied. He and his kind did succeed in destroying poor Hubert Humphrey in Chicago and electing Richard Nixon, a not inconsiderable historical accomplishment.

So it was worth trying to understand something about the New Left, just as it was worth trying to understand something about the Klan, and the black militants, and the army coffeehouses, and the draft dodgers, and such Newark figures as strong man Tony Imperiale and Kamiel Wadud, the Moslem leader, and why the South Bronx is being destroyed. Pete Young's unique talent, which I lack, is a talent

242

for making human contact with the alienated, the dissident, the angry, and the half mad, with all the diverse elements that make up subsurface America. He little knows of England who only England knows, and he little knows of America who knows only the halls of Congress, the offices of the upper bureaucracy, and the other Washington externals of the American political scene. For such reasons I am grateful to Pete Young and to his peculiar talent.

Monday, April 24—

There is a French word, *ennuyant,* for which, as with many French words, there is no precise English equivalent. It suggests boredom and annoyance and something else beside, a sort of weariness. What has been happening has been *ennuyant.*

I had a routine finger stick this morning, and then John gave me a physical examination. My hemoglobin was drifting lazily downward, and at some point, he said, he would have to give me a blood transfusion. He plans to maintain me at over 11 hemoglobin, so that I can continue to function while we wait to see what is really going on in my mysterious marrow. Then the readings came in, and they were low—low enough so that John decided I needed both a hemoglobin and a platelet transfusion.

I lunched with Rowly Evans and a co-founder of New York's Conservative Party, Kieran O'Doherty, an amusing, fast-talking fellow. I was rather appalled to find myself agreeing with some of the things he said—not many, but enough to make me nervous. Am I rapidly slipping to the right as my blood rapidly turns to water?

After I got back to the office, John called. He said I'd have the platelet transfusion this afternoon at five (I've just returned from it, as I write this, itchy from hives, but otherwise none the worse for wear) and a three-bag hemoglobin transfusion at two thirty tomorrow.

We talked a bit about the situation and what could be done about it. The diagnosis is still: ? But the doctors at NIH and outside specialists to whom they've shown the slides are more and more convinced that I have some form of marrow malignancy. "When we show your slides to someone who hasn't seen them before," said John (a bit ungrammatically), "they always shake their heads. They don't like the look of those cells. You remember Djerassi saying they looked very ugly. That's the way everybody reacts. But we don't know what they are." Thus I remain a medical mystery. A few months ago, I rather enjoyed being a mystery. Now it is *ennuyant*.

John talked about what drugs I might take if things got worse. He seems inclined to something called vincristine. The drug could be taken on an outpatient basis, intravenously. "Your hair would probably get thin, and you'd have a numbing of the ends of the fingers, but there are no really bad side effects." Somehow I hate the thought of losing my hair. Manly fellows are supposed to go bald early. Even so, I like having a fairly full head of hair.

John is very skeptical of steroids. They don't really get to the root of the trouble, he says, and although they make you feel full of beans for a while, you pay a very high price in side effects. This disappointed me. Remembering Jack Kennedy, who took steroids for adrenal insufficiency, I had envisaged myself filled with uncontrollable energy and horny as an old goat. But apparently Kennedy's were minimum maintenance doses; much bigger, more lethal doses are required for a malignancy.

Other possibilities are methotrexate—Djerassi's spe-

244

cialty is very heavy doses of methotrexate—POMP, a combination of four drugs; and L-asparaginase. The last is capable of attacking only the bad cells, and it got a big play in the press some time ago as a "cancer cure." But it is largely effective only against lymphoblastic leukemia, and it is also a very dangerous and quite often lethal drug.

The picture is complicated by the fact that the NIH doctors would be treating me for a disease they have not diagnosed. John says I will only be treated if the abnormal cells really begin to proliferate to the point where I can't be maintained by transfusions. But should I not then just let nature take its course and come to terms with Thanatos?

I think I'd do so if the only alternative were the laminar flow room. As it is, why not try drugs on an outpatient basis? One always grasps at straws. Too bad about the steroids, though. I'd have enjoyed one last fling of feeling horny as an old goat.

I begin to feel like Webster in T. S. Eliot—"Webster was much possessed by death / And saw the skull beneath the skin. . . . " The trouble is that death has begun to seem banal, boring. To die by inches is to die anticlimatically. I sense that other people are becoming almost as bored with my familiar old disease as I am. I find myself repeating the only line of the British paratroopers' song that I can remember: "Oh, gorblimey, wot an 'ell of w'y to die."

Gloomy. Maybe tomorrow, after I get three bags of good rich blood into my veins, I'll feel better.

Driving back from NIH, among the dogwood and flowering peach and the daffodils, I remembered one of my favorite lines. (A translation from the Greek—but by whom?): "The apple tree, the singing, and the gold." One of the loveliest lines in English. And the Washington April seems more lovely than ever. But how right T. S. Eliot was.

245

Thursday, April 27—

I had three bags of blood on Tuesday. It took about four hours. I spent the four hours on a cot in the clinic reading Malraux's conversation with de Gaulle, *Felled Oaks*. It was the same cot I'd had when I had my last transfusion, in September, just before the *dies gloriae*. There were two children having chemotherapy in the room when I came in, a little boy with thinning dark hair and a wasted little girl with a few strands of blond hair. Both were with their fathers—a nice Italian-looking man, and a Wasp-looking middle-aged man with a big stomach. Later, another little boy came in with his grandmother. When the doctor put in the needle, he began to scream, "Somebody hold my legs, somebody hold my legs."

All three had ALL, I suppose. There have been major advances in the treatment of lymphatic leukemia in children, and they have at least a chance to survive. But there is something intolerably unfair about leukemia's slaughter of the innocents, all the same. "Suffer little children to come unto me." But why?

About halfway through my second bag, a pretty blond woman came in and lay on the bed near the TV set, to get a bag of platelets. After a while, we chatted. I'd had a bag of platelets the day before, I said. What was her platelet count? Twenty-four thousand, she said. Mine had been twelve thousand, I said, topping her, but it was over forty thousand now.

"Aren't you Mr. Alsop?" she said. I said I was and asked her name. She told me and said she had been working for a Senator on the Hill and was still working, but only part time now. What was her diagnosis? I asked.

"AML," she said quietly. "What's yours?"

"I was diagnosed AML," I said, "but now they don't know what I have. How long since you were diagnosed?"

"Almost two years," she said. "I had a relapse in November, but I came back all right."

She left before my second bag was empty. I had an allergic reaction to my third bag. John gave me a Benadryl, and I went home and slept, and it went away.

This morning, the blond lady and I sat side by side in the clinic, with the rest of Nos Morituri Brigade, waiting for our finger sticks, and again we chatted briefly.

"I must say I don't enjoy this place," I said.

"Neither do I," she said. "Every time I come here, I look up at the building, and I say to myself, This is where I'm going to die."

Two years and a relapse, I thought. So far she's beaten the odds, but they're heavy odds. While she was having her finger stick, I looked at her carefully. Her hair seemed to be real; maybe it was a particularly skillful wig. There was also a strange quiet sweetness in her face. Was it always that way? Or only since she knew she had to die?

Malraux quotes de Gaulle as saying that the fall of France resulted from France's "inability to believe in anything at all." We are clearly infected with the same disease. It's a kind of political cancer.

Wednesday, May 3—

A queer day today. A marrow test at ten, then a date for lunch with Henry Kissinger and Joan Braden at the Sans Souci, then a column to write.

The marrow test was the worst ever. John had to go in several times before he got enough for a good reading. He

247

said he would call me after lunch, but I was already pretty sure what his news would be.

Lunch was agreeable. Joanie is always fun to be with, and Henry is a most witty and likable man. But his mood was somber, and with reason—ARVN seems to be crumbling in the North, and what may be crumbling with it is the whole elaborate Nixon-Kissinger structure of foreign policy. Like, to coin a phrase, a house of cards. The lunch was also professionally unrewarding. What I principally wanted to find out was the answer to this question: Why had the President nailed his colors to ARVN's shaky mast? Why, in other words, had he committed the prestige of the United States, and his own political future, to the dubious proposition that ARVN could defend South Vietnam? This is what he did in his televised speech, and again in his speech at the Connally ranch in Texas.

Why, for God's sake? Why not say, as he used to say, that he intended to fulfill his commitment to give the South Vietnamese a "reasonable chance" to defend themselves; that we would therefore provide them with all necessary logistic and air support; but that for the rest, as President Kennedy had said, it was their war, and they would have to win it for themselves? Surely to commit American prestige and his own to ARVN's military success was both dubious politics and dubious foreign policy.

Henry's answer was odd and unsatisfactory. He talked about bargaining power, and then he said something about my article about the President in a recent *Atlantic*. "Stewart, you got about twenty percent of the President in your article, which is better than most have done. But the answer to your question lies in the other eighty percent." Not very revealing.

I have a sense of foreboding. But I also have a sense that

something is in the works.* I decided to write a rather weak piece about McGovern rather than risk being caught out with a dated Vietnam piece.

After lunch, John called up. Much as I thought. Percentage of abnormal cells up to 44 percent or more. Hemoglobin wavering down below 13, since the transfusions; granulocytes at 300; platelets in the cellar at 16,000, and on the way down. John said he'd let me go to Avon for the division of the family property if I had a platelet transfusion before I went and if I promised to call him if I had any trouble. Meanwhile, he would give me more tests next week, then call a conference and decide whether to put me on some form of chemotherapy. What worried him most, he said, was that although I reacted well to the platelet transfusions, I couldn't hold the minimum platelet level. In all the slides from the marrow, they'd seen only one single megakaryocyte.

The thought of chemotherapy, after resisting it for so long, fills me with dread. Perhaps the steroids alone will somehow "goose"—John's words—the megakaryocytes back into action.

Driving home with Tish from NIH in the morning, I found various snips and snappets of memory running through my mind and jotted them down in my notebook. "I'll die tomorrow." (A novel? A movie? Can't place it.) "Enjoy, enjoy." (A book by Harry Golden, I think.) "Right back where we started from." (A line from a humorous poem? Again, I can't place it.) "And always keep a-hold of Nurse / For fear of finding something worse." (*Cautionary Tales*—the one about the boy who ran away from Nurse and was consumed by a lion. The nurse, in my case, is John Glick in particular and NIH in general.) "On pain of death,

* What was in the works was the blockade of Haiphong.

249

name not death to me. It is a word infinitely terrible." (John Webster—I think *The Duchess of Malfi.*)

On the way back to the house from NIH, we passed the Home for Incurables. It has always seemed to me a peculiarly cruel name for a hospital, and it seems especially so to me now.

Back home after work, I was annoyed to find that Andrew was out; he was visiting his Japanese girl friend, Kyo.

Andrew cheers me up as no one else can. He has developed a sort of special hop of his own, and I love to see his hop when he runs out to meet me. All little boys develop their own hop, I suppose, but Andrew's is very special.

I am too sentimental about children, especially my own, and especially the youngest. I suppose this may derive from my few drops of Roosevelt blood. T. R. was madly sentimental about his children. I remember the story about him sitting, an old fat man soon to die, on the porch at Oyster Bay, after his youngest son, Quentin, had been killed in France. He was rocking back and forth on a rocking chair, thinking he was alone, and repeating over and over again to himself, "Poor Quentie-quee. Poor Quentie-quee."

When I was young, I thought this story revoltingly sentimental. Now I understand it.

I think John Glick would understand it too. He adores Katie, his first-born, and he has been deeply worried about her. She had a fever some days ago, and it seemed that there was some possibility that she might have a potentially serious infection in her urinary tract. John was almost sure that the condition was temporary and without danger—but only almost sure. His Washington pediatrician proposed a diagnostic test. The procedure is almost without danger—but again, only almost.

At this point, all of a sudden, John ceased to be the crisp, self-assured, and knowledgeable Dr. Glick and became

a young father, worried to distraction. He would firmly decide to go ahead with the procedure, and then he would
decide equally firmly against it. Finally, to my amusement,
he asked old Dr. Alsop for his advice. I asked him if the test
was the only way to be absolutely sure that Katie had no
infection, and he said it was, and Dr. Alsop advised him to
go ahead and get it over with. He called a famous specialist
in New York, who gave him the same advice. He took it—
Katie was in fine shape. John was almost as euphoric as I was
in the days of the *dies gloriae*.

Tish and I fly to Hartford on Friday for the family con-
clave, to divide the furnishings of the Avon house and to
decide what to do about the property. Joe and Susan Mary
will be there, and John and Gussie, and Sis and Percy Chubb.
We're staying at John's house rather than in Wood Ford
Farm, for which I'm thankful. I'd hate the feeling of spending a last night in the house in which I grew up. I enjoy
my family, but I'm not looking forward to the weekend. The
occasion is a melancholy one, and I'm not feeling well—not
sick unto death, but uneasy, unwell.

Monday, May 8—

The Avon weekend was tolerable as long as we were
all pretty squiffed, which was a good deal of the time. But
it was somewhat intolerable in between times.

I went to Avon with a kind of mental window shade
drawn over my mind—no sentimental memories. But the
shade kept popping up, and I would see Ma exercising her
formidable forehand on the tennis court (now overgrown);
or holding out her arms to be bitten by the bees we children
would catch in the hollyhocks (bee stings were supposed to
be good for her arthritis); or talking and laughing in her
accustomed place before the fire in the living room, telling

her funny familiar stories with her funny familiar gestures.

Or I would catch a sudden glimpse, as the mental window shade popped up, of Pa in the front room, holding forth over the brandy and cigars ("If you don't like it here, why don't you go back to Russia?"); or venturing forth with his shotgun to shoot at cats and starlings (he hated cats and starlings); or telling stories about the Avon of old, when fat Mr. Sperry used to float down on his back from Avon to Simsbury on the Farmington River every Sunday, smoking a cigar and reading the Sunday papers; or when Mr. Ripley, who was First Selectman when Ma first came to Avon, gave Ma the big toe of his right foot in a bottle, when it had to be cut off, as a reward for her sympathy for his bunion.

I especially remembered Pa, who was First Selectman of Avon for thirty-three years, presiding with genial tyranny over the town meetings or the Republican caucuses in the old town hall, always with his hands in his back pants pockets. The Italians used to call him something that sounded like "Signor Gioffa." We children proudly thought it meant something like "The Big Chief." We learned later it just meant "Mr. Pockets."

I especially remembered Aggie Guthrie, who came to Avon at eighteen, when Joe was born in 1910, and nursed me through a sick childhood, and stayed till she died at seventy, of cancer. I remembered Aggie singing "Annie Laurie" and "I'll Take the High Road," and I remembered how, when I was scared, I would crawl into bed with her when I was really too old for such comforts.

Aggie had a broad Scots accent when she arrived—it got a little thinner with time—and since, when we were small children, we saw more of her than of our parents, when John and I went to school in Hartford we pronounced "moon" as "mun," and "bird" as "birrrd," which amused the other little boys. Aggie was a brilliant letter writer, though she never punctuated or capitalized. She wrote me much the best letters I got during the war. I saved them in the bottom of my trunk, as well as a lot of letters from some prewar girl friends. They all disappeared after I arrived back in Avon. I suspect Aggie disposed of them, because she didn't want Tish, whom she instantly took to, to see the girl friends' letters or hers.

I think Joe and Sis and John also had a mental window shade which kept popping up. Their manner was alternately excessively businesslike and oddly abstracted.

The Avon house, we agreed, is to be emptied of all objects, which will be divided equally between us, and then the house will be sold, if there are any takers, in a package deal with the rest of the real estate. It is no thing of beauty. The original house was built around 1830, and it is the basic Connecticut farmhouse—clapboard, low ceilings, narrow staircases. Pa simply added bits and pieces as the family grew, so that it is now big, comfortable, and utterly undistinguished—almost as undistinguished as my Washington house, but not quite.

Yet it is hard to wander about rooms in which you played as a little boy, which hardly have changed at all, and of which you have a mental map that can never be erased, and realize that it really is for the last time—that it's all over. We were smart enough to get a professional to appraise the contents and divide them into equal lots (except for Joe, who already has his share of the family loot and, according to John, a trifle more). We drew lots, and Tish and I got what everybody had agreed in advance was the bad lot. At least there was no bickering, and we are to get some objects I have always liked. But that is no compensation for the kind of breaking-up that the end of Avon symbolizes. This has been a tough year.

John Glick called me at the office this morning. This

253

afternoon, he said, there would be a meeting to decide what to do about me. I gather that the platelet problem is so serious that some form of chemotherapy is probably unavoidable.

Needwood
Sunday, May 14—

On Thursday, all the top specialists at NIH—Dr. Henderson, Dr. Carbone, Dr. Gralnick, and others, as well as John—had a morning meeting to decide on an Alsop diagnosis and an Alsop treatment. John called up about it in the afternoon, and we also talked about it at 5 P.M., when I went to NIH for a platelet transfusion.

The diagnosis is smoldering leukemia—smoldering, subacute, aleukemic leukemia. John said there had been only about a dozen cases under the same heading in the history of NIH. Therefore, treatment and prognosis were both difficult, the more so because my case was not exactly like any of the others.

Because I had had a near remission in the fall, John is hopeful that I will be especially responsive to drugs—in other words, that the bad cells will retreat more easily than usual. Moreover, the prognosis is certainly more hopeful than it would have been if I had had AML. Almost anything is more hopeful.

I am to have a marrow test on Wednesday, May 17 (my fifty-eighth birthday—nice birthday present), and if the bad cells are still increasing (which John obviously expects) I am to have a one-week course of steroids, tapering off thereafter. Most people react to steroids at first with euphoria, followed by depression when they are withdrawn. John Glick will try to control the depression by tapering off the

254

treatments. I think I'll be euphoric if the treatment works and depressed if it doesn't. But maybe that's too rational.

Somehow, it is a relief to get a diagnosis, however ambiguous, and to have the prospect of treatment, however chancey. Charlie Bartlett called on Friday, to inquire about the state of Alsop, and I asked him about Jack Kennedy's course of steroids. He said that Kennedy never talked about it, even to close friends (Charlie was one of the closest), but that he, Charlie, sensed when Kennedy had had a steroid treatment; "you could feel him sort of going into high gear."

Needwood
June 4—

A lot has happened since May 17, my fifty-eighth birthday, when I had my last marrow test, most of it bad.

My birthday test was good. John got spicules on the first try and, after his first look at the marrow, reported that the bad cells were "a bit down." The official report showed the proportion down from 42 percent to 24 percent, a sharp drop. John was doubtful, did a careful count himself, and confirmed the report. Before the May 17 marrow test, John and the other doctors had agreed that soon something would have to be done, though there was no firm agreement on what the something should be—steroids, chemotherapy, some immunological treatment. The May 17 marrow encouraged John's optimistic suspicion that my disease may be cyclic and that the up cycle (or down—depends on how you look at it) is now beginning.

Then we spent the weekend of May 20 at Needwood, and I suffered the Bluegill's Revenge.

As noted earlier, Father infected me with a mania for

shooting small birds with a shotgun and pulling small fish out of the water with a fly rod. As also noted earlier, I have always—and much more so since I got sick—had a faint feeling of ambivalence about killing these small living things. This is especially true of the birds, but I am even weak enough so that I sometimes get a faint sense of guilt about a fish, as it wriggles in my hand and stares at me with its unblinking eye. It has sometimes occurred to me that one day the thousands of small birds and small fish I have killed might get their revenge.

They got it the weekend of May 20. I went down to the pond at Needwood with my fly rod and pulled out about a dozen bluegills. They were barely big enough to eat, but I have a guilty compulsion to eat what I kill; otherwise I become in my own mind a killer-for-fun. So I cleaned the fish. I vaguely remember the sharp back fin of one bluegill pricking a finger on my right hand.

At the office on Tuesday, Amanda noticed an angry red spot on my finger and said she thought it looked infected. I had lunch with Djerassi at the Metropolitan Club—he was alternately fascinating and incomprehensible—and showed him the finger, and he said it looked "varry ogly," a favorite phrase. I went to NIH that afternoon for a platelet transfusion, and Dr. Miller—John was in California on a combined business and pleasure trip—took a swab from the finger. The next day I was back on the hated thirteenth floor of NIH, for a ten-day course of gentamicin. Thus did the ghosts of all those little fish—cheered on, no doubt, by the ghosts of great piles of little birds—get their revenge. It was a damned unpleasant revenge: chills, fever, platelet rejection, malaise, anorexia, two marrow tests, and other ills that man is heir to, including boredom and fear.

While I was in the hospital, I sensed that a debate was

256

going on about what to do with me. John was in California for most of my stay, so he couldn't take a direct part in the debate. I also sensed that there was considerable psychic pressure on Ed Henderson and the other doctors to do *something* about me. My white counts are dangerously low, and I can only hold a platelet transfusion for a couple of days—in the hospital, the platelet count went down twice under 5,000.

Part Three

AFTER I WROTE the sentence with
which the June 4 entry in my journal abruptly ends,
I had an experience most of us have had at one time or
another. I got bored with the sound of my own voice—or, in
this case, my own typewriter.

I used to have this experience rather regularly when I
was lecturing. During most of the sixties, all four of my
older children were in expensive schools or colleges, and I
had to find more money somewhere. So every year, in late
winter, when the bills were piling up, I would take off on
a two-week lecture tour. It was a grueling business—Albu-
querque one night, Salt Lake City the next, Los Angeles the
next, Cleveland the next, bad weather, planes that landed
at the wrong place, missed connections. But it was rewarding
in some ways.

It gave me a notion, though a faint one, of the vast
glandular energy required by a politician running for office.
It also gave me a notion of what most people were interested
in and what they were not.

In the early Kennedy era, for example, I learned to
count on several questions on the Peace Corps in the ques-
tion-and-answer period. I went to a party at the White

261

House in 1961, just back from a lecture tour, and President Kennedy asked a polite question about the tour. I remarked that everywhere I went I got questions about the Peace Corps.

"What do you say?" asked the President.

"I say I never thought the thing would work worth a damn, but it seems to be working pretty well," I said.

"Just what I think," he said.

The next year the questions were all about "managed news." In the early Johnson era, there were always questions about the Johnson personality—was he *really* like that? In the later Johnson era, especially at colleges, the questions were about Vietnam and the draft, of course.

I remember best the first question I was asked after the first lecture I ever made. This was in the town hall in Detroit after I'd come back from a month in the Soviet Union in 1955. I had described as best I could what life was like in Russia in those days, when the ghost of Josef Stalin still stalked the land. When I ended the lecture a lady with stiffly curled pearl-gray hair stood up and asked me angrily, "You mean those Russians are *socialistical?*"

"Yes, madam," I said, "they are socialistical." What else was there to say?

On my two-week tours, I would start out fresh with a semimemorized talk, and for the first week all would go well. But at some point during the second week, the same thing always happened to me. I would hear my own voice droning out the now overfamiliar words. Suddenly I would sense that I was boring the audience half to death. Worse, I was boring *myself* half to death.

That is precisely what happened to me when I wrote that sentence about my platelets being down to under 5,000. Suddenly I realized that no sensible reader of this book could fail to be bored by this sad little fact about my damned platelets, and, what was more, I was bored myself. So I stopped writing the journal.

After the episode of the Bluegill's Revenge I had some odd or interesting medical experiences, though, and I shall briefly recapitulate them.

I was right in suspecting that there was psychic pressure to do something about me. The gentamicin took care of the bluegill's infection, but the infection left me in bad shape. The percentage of abnormal cells in my marrow was over 40 percent again, and my counts were lousy; I had to have a platelet transfusion twice a week, meaning that my marrow was making hardly any platelets on its own. I was up and about, writing the column, playing tennis, spending pleasant summer weekends at Needwood. But I was skating on very thin ice all the same. The doctors knew it, of course, and by that time I knew enough about my disease to know it myself.

I had had no treatment at all, except for transfusions to maintain me, and by this time it was a year since I had been diagnosed. I used to joke with John Glick about what it would do to the reputation of the august NIH if I died and the fact came out that NIH had done nothing at all to treat my disease. He laughed, but I think it was not entirely a laughing matter to some of the other NIH doctors.

My new diagnosis, "smoldering" or "aleukemic" leukemia, was, I suspect, a way of saying that the doctors really didn't know just what was wrong. Doctors are unwilling to admit that they are puzzled—almost as unwilling as political writers. I enjoy irritating John Glick by pointing out that even the best doctors don't really know as much about the human body as a good political journalist knows about the body politic.

The question remained: What to do about Alsop? One doctor, who specialized in such operations, wanted to give me a marrow transplant, using my brother Joe as a donor. A marrow transplant is a nasty business. The marrow of the patient, both good cells and bad, is destroyed by chemical means or by irradiation. A large amount of marrow is withdrawn from a matched sibling—in this case, brother Joe— and injected into the veins of the patient.

The patient is of course in extreme danger while he is without a marrow, or while the new marrow is not functioning, or functioning only marginally. One chief threat to life is from infection, so at NIH, patients with marrow transplants are treated initially in laminar flow rooms. The other chief threat to life is from rejection—the body of the transplantee rejects the alien marrow, just as a transplanted heart or other organ is rejected.

The doctor who wanted to give me a marrow transplant came in to talk to me. My blood counts were improving a bit—a little bit—at this point, and my most recent marrow test showed no increase in the abnormal cells. I mentioned these small encouraging signs to the doctor, a brusque, unsympathetic type in his thirties.

"Let's forget about the numbers game," he said, with a hint of irritation in his tone. "It's time to face some facts."

The implication was that I would soon die if I didn't have a marrow transplant, though the doctor didn't exactly say so. I replied that I'd think it over and let him know what I decided. Thereafter my reportorial instincts reasserted themselves sufficiently to ask a couple of other doctors (John Glick was still in California at the time) about the results of marrow transplants in NIH up to that point.

There had been, it turned out, twelve transplants. The patients had all been young, mostly in their preteens to early twenties. Several had died in the laminar flow room, and those who survived the initial transplant lived, with one exception, only for a few miserable months, during which they were constantly sick almost unto death. The exception was a boy in his teens who was at that time still alive. But even he was plagued by infections and other disorders. Why, then, should this doctor want to do a transplant operation on a fifty-eight-year-old man with his sixty-one-year-old brother as a donor?

There are several possible explanations. One is that he had become genuinely convinced that I would die very soon without a transplant and that therefore the operation was justified *in extremis*. Another was simply that, like all specialists, he was eager to practice his specialty. A third and more cynical explanation was put forward by another doctor (not John), who clearly disliked him.

"Can't you see? He does a transplant on one well-known journalist with another well-known journalist as donor. It's a good story, picked up by the media. If you make it, fine; if you don't, you would have died anyway. Either way, it's a big plus for him."

My own guess is that the truth lies somewhere between explanations one and two. In any case, it was not difficult for me to decide firmly that, whatever happened, I would not have a marrow transplant.

Barring a transplant, there remained that question: What to do about Alsop? A course of chemotherapy in the laminar flow room was one possibility. But to this I was passionately opposed, and John Glick and Ed Henderson and most of the other doctors who were consulted also opposed chemotherapy. Chemotherapy is always dangerous, but with my low counts—especially the low granulocyte count—it would be doubly dangerous. For chemotherapy attacks the good cells as well as the bad, and I had very few good cells.

Finally, *faute de mieux*, a treatment John Glick candidly described to me as "highly experimental" was decided upon. By this time, John and the other doctors had agreed that the withdrawal of the allopurinol had not caused the near remission in the fall of the year before. Otherwise, they reasoned, the disease would not have reasserted itself. (I have never been able to follow this reasoning. It seems to me that the withdrawal of the allopurinol might have given the body a chance to fight back; that the body almost won the fight; but that the disease, stubborn like all cancers, hung on grimly and fought its way back. No doubt this is most unscientific.) In any case, John and the other doctors had come to believe that it was the mysterious September virus, rather than the withdrawal of the allopurinol, that had almost cured me.

Viremia has been known, though very rarely, to induce remissions by stimulating the body's natural resistance. Therefore, the doctors reasoned, why not induce in me a sort of controlled artificial viremia? The instrument was at hand, in a medication known as "Poly I:C." (For those who like to know such things, Poly I:C is a "synthetic, double-stranded RNA, polyriboinosinic-cytidylic acid.") Animal experiments had suggested, though inconclusively, that Poly I:C, injected into the veins, tended to reduce abnormal cells, and there had been a few cases in which Poly I:C injections appeared to have induced partial remissions in human leukemics, apparently by inducing in the marrow and the blood an antiviral agent called "interferon," which heightens resistance to the leukemic cells. The results of these experiments had been so inconclusive that they had been discontinued, but my case was so atypical, and the re-

266

mission after the September flu so suggestive, that it was decided to try me out on a course of Poly I:C.

It was an interesting experience (though, again, one could wish one were not so personally involved). After lunch on June 9, Tish drove me to NIH, and we took the elevator, slow and crowded as always, up to the thirteenth floor again. I got into bed, and John came in, stuck a needle into my right arm, and hooked me up to a bottle, about the size of a beer bottle, filled with what looked like plain water. It dripped into my veins in about forty minutes, and John removed the needle at 3 P.M. I felt nothing at all, for more than two hours. About half past five I began to feel a certain malaise. I was a bit chilly and asked for a blanket.

Just before six, I began to shiver, and by ten minutes past six, I was shaking so uncontrollably that the whole bed shook with me. I felt cold—colder than I have ever felt before, cold in the pit of my belly, cold to the very tips of my fingers and toes. Tish piled half a dozen heated blankets on top of me. Then the chill began to abate, and for about ten minutes I lay under my pile of blankets, luxuriating in the warmth. Then the warmth became altogether too warm, and I threw off the blankets. In a few minutes more my temperature shot up to 103, and sweat showed through my pajamas.

John was there, and he reassured me that all was as anticipated. Then I had another chill, even more violent, and after it my temperature went above 104. This second chill was not supposed to happen, and it seemed to me that John was looking just a bit nervous. But the fever had almost disappeared by midnight, and there were no more chills. I spent that night in the hospital. The next morning I felt well enough to eat a hearty breakfast and go to the office to work on a column.

That was the first day of a peculiar three-week routine. After lunch every Monday, Wednesday, and Friday, I would show up at NIH, take the Poly I:C into my veins, and wait for the chill and the fever. I never again had two chills, but I had one chill which was even more violent than those first two, and after it my temperature went over 105. That was the only time I was really scared. Toward the end of the course, the chills and fever were markedly milder, and by the next morning I always felt well enough to leave the hospital and go to work.

John had told me that the purpose of the treatment was to prod or shock my marrow into doing its cell-producing job again. I told him it sounded like trying to badger a lazy, sick old bird dog, who just wanted to doze by the fire, into getting out into the field looking for birds again. He said that was about right.

There were small signs that the bird dog was at least stirring in his sleep. My counts improved a bit, and when John did a marrow test after the course, the percentage of bad cells was under thirty, for the first time in a good many weeks. But after a few more weeks, the bird dog snoozed again; the counts went back down to where they had been. John decided on a second course of Poly I:C.

During the first course I had managed to go on writing the column for *Newsweek*, but it seemed to me the quality had dropped off, and I hate writing a bad column and hate even more reading a bad column I have written. So with the kind concurrence of the *Newsweek* editors, I dropped the column during my second three-week course of Poly I:C.

After the second course, my marrow was again under 30 percent abnormal, and the counts were a bit better. But it was clear that the Poly I:C had not induced the hoped-for remission. No one knows, or ever will know, whether those

268

chills and fevers did me any good—perhaps they did. At least they did me no harm.

The experience was, as noted earlier, interesting in its own peculiar way. I became entirely accustomed to it and could have endured it more or less indefinitely, although I was thoroughly glad when it was over. The chills, which always lasted between thirty and fifty minutes, reminded me of the experience of flying in an airplane during very stormy weather. You know the trip will end, and you are sure—well, almost sure—that it will end happily. Meanwhile, you dislike it very much indeed, and the time seems to crawl by. Then the plane breaks through the heavy clouds, and there are the lights of the airfield below, and you sigh with relief—just the feeling I had when the shaking began to abate and the delicious warmth began to creep back into my body.

By September, with the Poly I:C treatment behind me, I felt well enough to get on about the business of living, and I was fully operational again. Henry Kissinger was scheduled to make a trip to Moscow, to wrap up the details of the agreements reached during the Nixon-Brezhnev talks in late spring. Kissinger is a sort of intermittent friend of mine. He has occasionally been infuriated by something I have written—he was particularly annoyed by a column to the effect that a "Kissingerless Nixon filled with hubris" might be a receipt for disaster—but most of the time we are friends.

He is a good friend. Kissinger can be very tough, as some of his subordinates gladly attest. But there is also a thoughtfulness about him—one is almost tempted to use the word "sweetness"—that is endearing and that perhaps helps to account for his success with the ladies.

Henry asked for a résumé of my case to take with him

269

to Russia; perhaps the Russians, who had made important advances in the treatment of leukemia, would have some brilliant new ideas for treating me. At first I thought he was just being polite, but he kept insisting. Finally John Glick agreed to write a memorandum summarizing my case. For any doctor reader who might be interested in a technically accurate account, John's memorandum is included in an appendix. The Russian response Henry brought back with him is also included in the appendix. It is almost laughably ambiguous, saying, in effect, that NIH had done just the right thing.

It seemed oddly naïve of Henry Kissinger to suppose that the Russians would risk proposing some bold new treatment for his journalistic friend; if I promptly died, always a possibility, it could only make trouble. But Henry told me that the high-level official who gave him the memorandum volunteered that they had treated cases similar to mine at the Soviet Oncology Institute and that several of these cases had remained stable for a long time—in one instance, for ten years.

John Glick says my marrow slides have become positively boring. Each slide looks like the last, and the abnormal cells, still unidentifiable, look tediously the same. He too now speculates that this stable condition might last for years—conceivably even for ten years.

I find that I am oddly ambivalent about this possibility. When I began to write this book, I accepted John's odds, 20 to 1 against more than two years of life. Suppose I last much longer? I can imagine rude whispered comments: "Isn't that old creep the man who wrote a book about how he was dying of cancer?" Curious, the prospect of being embarrassed to be still alive.

To a leukemic who has got used to thinking as a leukemic, ten years is a very long time. I think I would be willing to settle for considerably less, as long as the exit is quick, sudden, and painless. If I survive, I shall be sixty in May 1974. Sir William Osler once remarked that it might be a good idea to chloroform everybody on his or her sixtieth birthday. After sixty the trail is all downhill. In fact, chloroform might be appropriate as soon as a person has to wear reading glasses; that is where the downhill trail really starts.

Meanwhile, I am glad that I am still able to write a column, play tennis, and enjoy life. For months now, a pleasant young man who does not want his real name used—call him Bob Park—has made it possible for me to do these things. Bob Park may have saved my life. He certainly made life a lot more pleasant for my brother Joe. To understand why, it is necessary for me to say more about platelets.

One of the reasons John and the other doctors decided they had to do *something* about patient Alsop was that my damned platelets were in such awful shape. They tried several donors, but none of them gave me what is known in the trade as "a good increment." My platelet count would rise only to the modest level of 30,000 or so, and in three or four days the count would sink sadly down far below the 20,000 danger point and I would have to have another platelet transfusion. Then in June, Dr. Ron Yankee, a very able platelet specialist who then headed the "plasma pharesis laboratory" where platelet transfusions are prepared, discovered Bob Park.

When I first began to try to understand the basic facts about leukemia, I had gathered from John Glick that the only danger from platelet transfusions was from hepatitis —that if a patient was lucky enough not to get hepatitis, transfusions could continue indefinitely. But nothing is simple about leukemia. For one thing, producing the small plas-

271

tic bag of platelets that will keep a leukemic alive for a few days is not a simple matter. It requires hours of work and a lot of professional expertise. It is also a long, boring business for the donor.

The donor sits in a high reclining chair with a needle in his arm for upwards of three hours. Four large plastic bags of blood are withdrawn from his body by simple gravity; the bags are held below the level of his arm. An elaborate machine separates the platelets from the four bags by a centrifugal process, and the blood, now *sans* platelets, is reinserted in his body, again by gravity; the bags are held above the level of his arm. A healthy marrow quickly replaces the missing platelets in the donor's blood.

The platelets withdrawn from the donor's body are then "resedimented." The bag of pinkish stuff that has been withdrawn from the donor is put in an upright plastic test tube. The hemoglobin is heavier than the platelets, and it drifts gently, over a period of several hours, to the bottom of the tube. The platelets, now almost pure, are withdrawn from the top of the tube.

This is done so that a donor can give platelets to a patient with a wholly different blood type. If the hemoglobin were not removed, the recipient would have a reaction, perhaps a violent one, and the blood and platelets would both be rejected by the body's immune response mechanism. The end result of all this trouble is a small plastic bag of a yellowish milky fluid, still with a faint trace of pink. The bag is transfused, again by gravity, into the leukemic's blood stream, and thus he is permitted to go on living for a few days more.

How does the patient feel when his platelets are low? John Glick and I have had a running argument on this score. He claims that there is no symptom of low platelets, other than bleeding or petechiae, that a patient is capable of sensing, and I tell him that he says this only because he has never had low platelets.

I have never had a serious hemorrhage, though my platelets have been very low indeed on several occasions. But I have had nosebleeds which refused to stop for several hours. One of the small unpleasant habits a leukemic acquires is to glance always at his handkerchief after he blows his nose, hoping not to see the telltale traces of blood. John Glick tells me to blow my nose gently, with my mouth and throat open, but I maintain this is physically impossible.

I have also had petechiae. These are small hemorrhages beneath the skin. A leukemic learns to look for these small red spots on his skin or on the roof of his mouth, for they are sure warnings that a transfusion is needed soon.

The petechiae are entirely painless, and there is no sure sign that a nosebleed is coming. But when my platelets are very low I feel a sort of malaise. The French have a phrase: *Je me sens bien dans ma peau*—"I feel well in my skin." When my platelets are low, I do not feel well in my skin. I can usually make a pretty accurate guess at my platelet level, and not only by counting the days since my last transfusion. When my platelets are really low—10,000 or under—I do not feel at all well in my skin. There is a constant sense of uneasiness.

Until recently, leukemics with a low platelet count were transfused with "random platelets," as I was originally. Platelet transfusion itself is a technique developed only within the last ten years or so. Dr. Djerassi was a chief inventor of the technique—he received a Mary Lasker Award for his work. But there is one trouble with using platelets from any random donor. Almost always, transfusions can continue for only a couple of months. By that time, the recipient has developed antibodies. His white cells have come to recognize the transfused cells as alien to the body, and they fight and kill the life-giving invaders.

This is where HL-A matching—and Bob Park—come in. Again, for those who like technical terms, HL-A is an abbreviation for the "human leukocyte-locus A," whatever that means. The point is that everybody inherits two HL-A antigens from his mother and two from his father.

The technique of typing and matching these antigens in the blood is new—Dr. Ron Yankee, until recently the platelet specialist at NIH, had a lot to do with perfecting it, starting in the late sixties. The work has been carried on by Dr. Robert Graw. If it were not for Dr. Yankee and Dr. Graw and their platelet laboratory, I might not be alive at all. I certainly would not be playing tennis or writing a column.

That I am still doing both is largely due to Bob Park, a technician with NIH and—quite aside from his lovely platelets—a very nice man. Bob's HL-A antigens are not a perfect match for mine. As they have been identified, the antigens have been given numbers. Mine are 10 and 12, from one parent, and 3 and 50, from the other. Bob's are 3 and 50, and 10 and 18. Theoretically, my body ought to make antibodies to fight that number 18 antigen, which I don't have. For mysterious reasons, it never has, and my "increments" from a transfusion by Bob have actually increased, rather than the other way about.

As this suggests, there are still unraveled mysteries about the business of platelet matching. Ron Yankee found a lady employee of NIH who was a perfect match—10, 12, 3, 50—and he and John were confident that my blood would happily accept her platelets. Instead, I reacted with hives and an almost total rejection; there was hardly any incre-

274

ment at all. My brother Joe, whose antigens are, like the lady's, a carbon copy of mine, bravely stood in three times for Bob when Bob went on vacation in August 1972, and I had a good increment every time. But given Joe's age, and some indications of heart irregularity, John Glick does not want to use Joe as donor any more than necessary.

He and Ron Yankee tried several other donors with close antigen matches, but my response was always the same —hives and partial rejection. Once John tried a transfusion from my son Joe, but within an hour of the transfusion I was liberally spotted with hives and got a very modest increment. Finally John tried my third son, Stewart, who has Bob Park's antigens in reverse—10, 18, and 3, 50. Stewart spent four hungry hours (he had forgotten breakfast) in the donor's chair on the day after Christmas, December 26, 1972, and I had my transfusion at about seven o'clock that evening.

The next morning I had a finger stick, and John Glick called me at the *Newsweek* office a couple of hours later. "It worked," he said exultantly. Stewart's platelets had given me a nice healthy increment, from under 20,000 platelets to over 42,000. Not quite as good as Bob Park, but good enough.

It was a nice post-Christmas present. Bob Park is young and healthy. He has no intention of leaving NIH, and in an emergency there's always brother Joe as a backup. But it is a nervous feeling, all the same, to live from week to week dependent for life itself on the cells in another man's blood. It is nice to have Stewart as another backup.

Thirteen-year-old Nicky's blood is a carbon copy of Stewart's, as Joe's is of mine. John Glick was sure that Nicky would also be a good backup in an emergency, and one day in January, Nicky, accompanied by Tish for moral support, went to the third floor of the east wing, got into the reclining chair, and, his eyes tight closed and his belly empty (he had been too scared to eat breakfast, he said), held out his arm for the needle. It hardly hurt at all, he said later, but about halfway through the process he had a reaction—he turned light green and complained of feeling sick. The platelets were resedimented for four hours, but they looked suspiciously pinkish when I had my transfusion that afternoon. The next morning John called up to say that Nicky's platelets hadn't worked; there was no increment at all. Perhaps Nicky's reaction accounted for the failure. Of course I didn't tell Nicky that his platelets hadn't helped.

At one point another bureaucratic ruling was promulgated—no one seemed to know by whom or for what purpose—that no donor should give platelets more than twenty times in one year. That would have ruled out Bob Park, who had already given me more than twenty donations, and made me wholly dependent on brother Joe's elderly platelets. It would have been a real strain on Joe's heart for him to sustain me all by himself. Fortunately, strings were pulled and an exception made.

One doctor bureaucrat, I was told, proposed that the whole expensive platelet-matching operation be abandoned entirely. This, he argued, would not only save money, it would be medically significant. It would be interesting to see how many patients survived without transfusions, or with random platelet transfusions only, and for how long.

Actually, this proposal was not quite as brutally irrational as it may seem. In medicine, as in other fields, cost has to be weighed against effectiveness. Theoretically, it would be possible to find a perfect HL-A matched platelet donor for every leukemic in need of platelets—for example, as one doctor at NIH proposed, all the members of the armed services could be HL-A typed. But leukemia is a relatively rare disease, and leukemics who need platelets regularly are decidedly bad insurance risks anyway. To ensure matched platelets for every leukemic who needed them would require a vast expansion of laboratory facilities and a disproportionate investment in time and inconvenience on the part of the donors, all to prolong the lives of a relative handful of patients likely to die soon in any case. At least in Pentagonian cost-effectiveness terms, the results would not justify the expense.

As I have seen more and more of NIH, I have been reminded increasingly that the place is, after all, a government bureaucracy, and not at all immune to Parkinson's law and the other abuses to which all bureaucracies are heir. And yet I owe a lot to NIH and to the people who inhabit the place. For one thing, I owe NIH my life, which NIH has saved, or at least prolonged, repeatedly. In October 1972, NIH performed this lifesaving function once again. While my life was being saved, I had an experience that haunts me still.

On Friday, October 13, playing tennis in the late afternoon, I began to feel a rawness in my chest. I finished the tennis game and climbed up to the house to change for dinner at Kay Graham's. I felt, I told Tish, a bit rocky, but not rocky enough to beg off the dinner date. The dinner was small, the food delicious, and the conversation—mostly about the Watergate affair—interesting. But by ten o'clock I knew something was wrong. I felt cold, and I began to shiver gently. We made our excuses, and I asked Tish to take the wheel for the drive home. By the time I got home, I was having a severe chill. I got into bed, pulled up the covers, and Tish took my temperature—it was just over 100. Not enough to worry about, I thought.

277

The next day I was back in the same room I had occupied more than a year before, when I had first been admitted to NIH. I had lobar pneumonia, and John Glick had hooked me up to the familiar I.V. Two bottles of antibiotics dripped alternately into my veins. This time, I had the privileged bed beside the window, and the bed near the door was occupied by a muscular young man with brown skin, curly black hair, and a huge grin.

His name was odd—Lekoj Anjain. He was, it turned out, from the Marshall Islands. He had been a one-year-old baby in 1954, when we Americans tested our first deliverable hydrogen bomb on Bikini, one of the Marshalls.

As it happened, I knew a good deal about the Bikini bomb. With the help of Dr. Ralph Lapp, an atomic scientist who used to act as my mentor in such matters, I had done a lot of reporting on it. So had brother Joe. As a result, Joe and I were the first to describe, in our joint column, the phenomenon of nuclear fallout.

The Bikini bomb was much more powerful than Edward Teller and the other scientists in charge had anticipated. Moreover, it had an unanticipated effect. It churned up great mounds of earth below the explosion point. The earth was turned into light dust by the force of the explosion. This heavily irradiated dust followed the wind patterns until it fell out of the skies. Some of it fell on the *Lucky Dragon,* a Japanese trawler more than ninety miles from the explosion point. The members of the crew all suffered from radiation sickness, but none of them, so far as is known, died from leukemia.

The fallout also filtered down on others of the Marshall Islands, including the island of Rongelap more than one hundred miles from Bikini. Inhabitants of these islands also took a dose of radiation. Rongelap was Lekoj Anjain's native island.

278

I am still haunted by a mental image of Lekoj as a cheerful brown baby playing in the sand under the palm trees of Rongelap, as the sky lit up above him from the great explosion on Bikini, and playing still, feeling no harm, as the dust of the fallout settled around him. The cheerful brown baby was now my roommate, nineteen-year-old Lekoj, and he had, John Glick told me, a particularly vicious variety of acute myelogenous leukemia.

There was no doubt at all that the bomb and the leukemia were cause and effect. The Nagasaki and Hiroshima bombs had induced leukemia in a good many Japanese. Several inhabitants of the Marshall Islands had developed suspicious lymph nodes as a result of the Bikini test. But Lekoj was the first case of leukemia from the fallout of a hydrogen bomb test.

The Atomic Energy Commission had flown his father out from Rongelap to be with him. His father was a tough-looking little man, much smaller than Lekoj. For hours at a time he would sit by Lekoj's bedside, saying nothing at all. Once in a long while he would reach out and touch Lekoj's hand, and sometimes Lekoj would mutter something, in Marshallese, and grin.

Lekoj spoke hardly any English, so there was not much communication between us. Every morning I would smile, and he would grin back—his teeth were perfect—and I would ask, "How you feel?"

Usually he would reply, "Fine. Fine." But toward the end of the twelve days we spent together, he would be more likely to say, still with a grin, "No good. Feel deezy." He was being given very powerful chemicals, in an attempt to induce a remission, and he was nauseated. But he remained remarkably cheerful. I wondered if he knew how sick he was.

He was a heavily built young man, and his muscles rippled under his skin. But there was a curiously gentle

279

quality about him, a softness, a kind of endearing childishness—it was very easy to imagine him as that baby in the sand under the sudden glare of light.

Despite the lack of a common tongue, we had our common sickness. One morning Lekoj was taken to the operating room for a marrow test, and when he came back I asked, "Marrow hurt bad?"

He replied enthusiastically, "Marrow hurt *bad*." Then I had a marrow, and the same exchange took place in reverse.

We both had a hemoglobin transfusion on the same day. I said, "Blood make you feel good."

He enthusiastically agreed again. "Yes, blood feel *good*."

On October 27, at long last, John took the needle out of my arm and pronounced the pneumonia under control. I asked Lekoj how he felt for one last time, and this time he said again, "Fine. Fine." We said good-bye, and I left the hospital.

With Lekoj's permission, I had written a column about him. I imagine it was because of the column that someone in the Interior Department, under whose bureaucratic aegis Lekoj fell, called Amanda in the office about ten days after I had left the hospital and asked her to tell me that Lekoj was dead.

Amanda hated to tell me, but finally she did.

"What did he die of?" I asked.

"The man said pneumonia," she said, and then quickly added, "But don't you go thinking it was your fault."

The chances are that Lekoj picked up whatever virus or bacteria had made me sick. But John Glick told me not to worry, that the chemotherapy had failed and poor Lekoj was terminal anyway.

Lekoj's death deeply depressed me for a while. There

was, of course, what might be called the send-not-to-ask syndrome. With my low defenses the pneumonia might well have killed me; John Glick was surprised by how quickly I recovered, given my corporal's guard of granulocytes.

There was also the depressing feeling, hard to shake off, that I had somehow been responsible for Lekoj's death. There was the further feeling, as hard to shake off, that we Americans were responsible for his death—that we had killed him with our bomb. His was the world's first death from a hydrogen bomb, and the bomb was ours. And finally, there was the feeling of the desperate, irrational unfairness of the death of this gentle, oddly innocent young man. For some time, I found a line, I think from T. S. Eliot (though I can't find it), going through my mind: "The notion of some infinitely gentle / Infinitely suffering thing."

Before Lekoj died, I had long believed in my mind that the nuclear weapon, in its indiscriminate, unimaginable brutality, was an insane weapon, suicidal, inherently unusable. Now I knew it in my heart.

AT THE START of this peculiar book, I remarked that when I found myself on top of the dump at Needwood, gasping like a beached fish, it was the second time I had said to myself, "Face it, Alsop. You're in trouble." One way to end this book is to recall that other time—it was in the summer of 1944—when I first had to face the fact that I was in trouble.

I served in Italy with the King's Royal Rifle Corps as an infantry platoon commander for several months in late 1943. It was not an experience I found at all enjoyable, for reasons that anyone who has ever served in the infantry will understand. One day in December 1943, my cousin Ted Roosevelt, a brigadier general in the U.S. Army, appeared at battalion headquarters. (He stopped his jeep in a whirl of dust, thus inviting, and getting, shellfire from the Germans, which did not make him popular.) He told me that it was about time to get into my own army, and I agreed. George Thomson, who was in the same battalion, also wanted to transfer to the American army. Ted Roosevelt wrote a To Whom It May Concern note, recommending us for transfer into his old division, the First. Armed with this note and another from our battalion's commanding officer, George and I set off for General Eisenhower's SHAEF headquarters in Algiers.

We proudly produced our handwritten notes for perusal by a colonel in charge of personnel in Algiers. "Jesus Christ," he muttered, "you two guys sure as hell are out of channels." Then he leafed through great mounds of papers in quadruplicate.

"Either of you guys happen to be a veterinarian?" he asked.

We both shook our heads. He leafed through some more papers.

"You're not Methodist ministers, by any chance?" he asked.

Again we shook our heads.

"Sorry," he said. "We got slots for a veterinarian and a Methodist minister. Other than that, the orders are no more transfers of American citizens from foreign armies. Orders straight from Washington. Sorry."

George Thomson and I thus found ourselves in a most peculiar situation, a kind of military limbo. The King's Royal Rifle Corps was over-officered, and as soon as we left Italy our old platoons had been taken over by other officers. To return to our battalion as "supernumeraries" would have been most shaming, and besides, George and I agreed, there must be some better way of making a living than getting shot at all the time for $42 a month, then a British subaltern's pay.

I suppose in the American army we would have been sent to a Replacement Depot, or Repple Depple, but the British army, a much more casual organization, didn't work that way. If you were a "supernumerary"—an unemployed officer—you were expected to shift for yourself, find a spot somewhere, if possible with your own regiment.

George and I rented a double bedroom in a French lady's house and began to sniff around. The Americans would have none of us, though we tried again. All the KRRC battalions were overmanned. We got our regular pay, and a whisky allowance, and at first it was like a fine free leave. But after about a month, we were getting a bit desperate. We obviously couldn't wander about in this limbo forever. Then one evening in the Club Interallié, George Thomson, who was very good at running into people, ran into Lady Hermione Ranfurley, an aide and confidante of General Jumbo Wilson, the British general who was second in command under Ike.

George described our desperate situation to Lady Hermione, and she offered to wangle us into "quite a good parachute outfit—behind the lines, *coup de main,* all that sort of thing." It was run, she said, by an old friend of hers, a Colonel Sterling. The outfit, called the Special Air Services, or SAS, consisted of a couple of battalions, each commanded by one of the Sterling brothers, both of the Scots Guards. So, with an assist from Lady Hermione, we joined the SAS.

The SAS was quite different from the King's Royal Rifle Corps. The KRRC was respectable upper middle class, with approximately one Lord and two or three Hons (younger sons) per battalion. The SAS was full of Lords and Hons. Most of the officers were in the Guards (the snobbiest of the British regiments), and most of them seemed to belong to White's Club.

They were an eccentric lot. Colonel Sterling had a thing about hats. We all wore our regimental insignia on our hats. (In the British army, your regiment—and thus your approximate position in the social pecking order—was immediately distinguishable from your headgear.) Then somebody in London promulgated an order that all combat parachutists without exception were to wear pink berets and pink berets only. To Colonel Sterling the pink berets were as a red rag to a bull. The thought of discarding his Scots Guards peaked

284

cap and substituting "a horrible pink beret" was utterly abhorrent to him. So he flew off to London to persuade his
friend Winston Churchill to rescind the order.

In the end he succeeded, but in his absence, discipline,
which had been pretty loose before he left, became looser
still. Training consisted largely of a Guards-style battalion
parade at the sensible hour of ten in the morning, after
which the officers would retire to the officers' mess to drink
Algerian brandy.

When time hung heavy on their hands, the officers
would agree that it was time to have a bash. They would
call a nearby American fighter squadron and invite all those
interested over for the bash. The American pilots and the
British parachutists would drink copious drafts of Algerian
brandy, in a spirit of international amity, and then the bash
would begin, a tremendous Anglo-American brawl raging all
over the officers' mess. This custom was a bit embarrassing
to George Thomson and myself, partly because we didn't
enjoy brawling as much as the other participants seemed
to, and partly because we didn't know which side we ought
to join.

When we got our orders to sail back to England, in the
late winter of 1944, some of the White's Club members ar-
ranged to smuggle large quantities of Algerian brandy into
England. Their method was simple. They discarded the contents of a great many wooden boxes marked "Company
Stores" and packed them with brandy. They made a lot of
money; they bought the brandy for about 50 cents a bottle
and sold it for $5 or more, and at the same time, by their own
lights, they benefited suffering humanity—by that time London was terribly short of any kind of alcoholic beverage.

We arrived in Scotland, where SAS had a base, in April,
and George and I immediately applied for London leave—

I intended to pursue Tish, and George intended to pursue pleasure. During his pursuit of pleasure, in Rosa Lewis's Cavendish Hotel (which used to be a very good place to pursue pleasure), George again ran into somebody useful—in this case Hod Fuller, a handsome and dashing U.S. Marine lieutenant colonel in an outfit called the Jedburghs.

Hod Fuller suggested that we transfer from the SAS to the Jedburghs. Operation Jedburgh, he explained, was run jointly by the Allied secret services. The mission of the Jeds, he said, was to provide arms and liaison for the French maquis. To that end, Jed teams consisting of one American or English officer, one French officer, and a radio operator were to parachute into occupied France, where they would join maquis resistance groups.

Partly because we hankered to be with Americans again, George and I eagerly agreed to Hod Fuller's suggestion, and with help from him we ended up with the Jedburghs. (Hod Fuller's suggestion may have saved my life, since the SAS squadron to which I belonged was badly cut up in France.) The American Jeds were an interesting and uninhibited lot. They played poker for enormous stakes and swore a great deal, and they were as randy as young goats. They had one curious custom that astonished the English and the French.

The rather stiff British colonel who ran the Jedburgh base camp, at a handsome pile called Milton Hall, scheduled speakers once or twice a week. Often the speakers were experienced behind-the-lines operatives, and they were heard with respectful attention. But occasionally they were pompous blimps or officious civilians in uniform. I was first exposed to the curious custom of the American Jedburghs when an American OSS man—one of those of whom it was said that "OSS was the last refuge of the well connected"— made a long, self-important, and tedious speech.

"I wish with all my heart," he said, "that I could be with you boys in the field, but direct orders from General Donovan keep me, unfortunately, chained to my desk."

An American Jed in the back of the room murmured, "Fifty-five."

Another followed, more loudly: "Fifty-six."

In a rising crescendo, the American Jeds all shouted, "Fifty-seven, fifty-eight, *fifty-nine*, BULLSHIT!"

The OSS man retreated in confusion, while the Americans laughed and the more circumspect and better-disciplined French and British looked on in mixed admiration and amusement. Toward the end of the training period, the French and British would join in the chant.

I took an eight-jump parachute course in May and found a French partner, a big, handsome, brown-eyed St. Cyr captain whose *nom de guerre* was Richard Thouville —as René de la Tousche, his real name, he is still a good friend. Together we enlisted an American radio operator, nineteen-year-old Norman Franklin, who was a whiz with Morse code. The Jedburghs were generous about leaves and I pursued Tish assiduously, successfully enough so that by May her parents had agreed in principle to our getting married, although she was only eighteen. In early June, just before D-Day, Thouville hurt his ankle in a motorcycle accident, which meant that we couldn't jump into France for at least two weeks.

That evening, after a couple of whiskies, I telephoned Tish at her parents' flat on Pont Street and suggested that we get married right away, while Thouville was *hors de combat*. I thought there was very little chance that Mr. and Mrs. Hankey would agree—after all, my future was uncertain, and Tish was only eighteen. I could hear Tish arguing with them, as I put sixpence after sixpence into the pay telephone

287

in the officers' mess at Milton Hall. Tish is strong-minded, and she prevailed.

"Mummy and Daddy say we can get married Tuesday," she said into the telephone. I was astonished.

"Jesus Christ," I heard myself saying. "Trapped like a rat."

Despite this tactlessness, we were duly married on June 20, with George Thomson as best man. It had previously been impossible to get a hotel room anywhere in London, but the buzz bombs started just before we were married. Armed with a check for $1,000 from brother-in-law Percy Chubb, I hired a magnificent suite on the top floor of the Ritz for our honeymoon. The Ritz, like every other hotel, had emptied swiftly after the buzz bombs started.

We had a notably gregarious honeymoon. My brother John had come to England as a military policeman, but when he learned what I was up to, he quickly decided to become a behind-the-lines parachutist, too, and volunteered for OSS. He had been taking a parachute course when Tish and I were married, but he came to London a day or so later to stay at the Cavendish. Liquor was available in unlimited quantities at the Ritz—at four pounds, or $16, per bottle, but Percy Chubb's check took care of that. A continuous revel went on in our honeymoon suite, attended by John, George Thomson, Reeve Schley (who jumped into France with John), Rosa Lewis of the Cavendish, Rosa's Scottie dog, Kippy, and assorted eccentric Cavendish guests.

At one point Tish rather timidly asked whether we couldn't have one evening alone. The question amazed me.

"Good God, woman," I said. "Don't you realize I'm on leave?" There are those who wonder how Tish has put up with me all these years.

When our honeymoon ended, Thouville's foot had healed, and we were put on standby alert. The ranks began to thin at Milton Hall, as teams were sent into France, and discipline became virtually nonexistent. I went AWOL to London every weekend to see Tish, with my shaving kit and a change of shirts in my gas mask pack. We stayed at the Cavendish—Rosa Lewis adored Tish and kept giving her half-dead flowers—and once, when I'd had a remittance from Pa, at the Ritz again.

In mid-July, Jed Team Alexander—Thouville, Franklin, and myself—was put on full alert, and we left Milton Hall for London, to be ready to go on a couple of hours' notice. By special dispensation, as a newly married man, I was allowed to stay at the Cavendish with Tish. Three times in a row, we were told to be ready to jump that night. I would say a fond farewell to Tish and board a bus for the Special Ops airfield outside London, only to be told that the operation was canceled for that night.

Twice the weather was wrong. Once the "reception committee," the maquis group whose job it was to light fires in a prearranged pattern to guide our plane to the Drop Zone—Dee Zed in British military parlance—warned that there were Germans in the area. Each time Team Alexander returned dejectedly to London by bus. "Well, here I am again," I would tell Tish, as I crawled into bed with her at two or three in the morning.

By this time we had been thoroughly briefed on our mission. We were to be dropped with an O-group—*coup de main* specialists, whose mission was to blow up an important bridge—to a well-established maquis in the area of Aubusson and Guéret in central France. The towns were held by the Germans, but they were lightly held; this was before the breakthrough at Avranches, and most of the German troops were, of course, on the Normandy front. The countryside was maquis territory.

I had applied repeatedly for a transfer to the U.S. Army,

and after the third false alarm my transfer at last came through, no doubt as a result of Mother's little chat with Franklin Roosevelt. I borrowed a uniform from brother John. It fitted badly—John is shorter and broader than I am— and it was not nearly as dashing as my KRRC uniform. Moreover, I had just proudly put up my third pip—I had been made a temporary acting captain in the British army—and the transfer came through for Lieutenant Alsop. I consoled myself with the thought that an American lieutenant's pay was about three times a British captain's.

When we were alerted for the fourth time, Tish went with me in a taxi to the bus station. The first time I had kissed her good-bye rather emotionally, but after three false alarms I was carefully casual. "See you around two at the Cav," I said. As soon as I boarded the bus, I knew that this night we would jump. Thouville and Franklin and the O-group were on the bus, and the word had been passed that tonight we had a definite green light.

At the airfield, the situation was normal—nobody knew just who we were or where we were going or what plane we were going on. But we were finally trussed into our jump suits, complete with a slung carbine and an entrenching tool for burying our parachutes, and bundled into a plane, one of a flight of three bound for central France. On our plane a last-minute crisis occurred—the jump master assigned to our drop was nowhere to be found. An R.A.F. corporal was hastily assigned to act as jump master, and we took off with a roar. It was a bright moonlight night in midsummer.

As we crossed over the Normandy battlefield, the plane began to buck wildly and there were loud banging noises and great flashes of light. I thought for a moment we had hit a thunderstorm, but then I realized that the Germans were shooting at us. I glanced round the dimly lit plane and saw that, in a futile but instinctive gesture, every man had his hands clasped protectively over his crotch.

The flak stopped and we droned on through the night, over occupied France. The word was passed back from the cockpit that we had lost contact with the other two planes because of the antiaircraft fire. The pilot had been ordered to follow the lead plane, but with the help of his navigator he would try to find the Dee Zed on his own.

After about an hour of flying, the R.A.F. corporal who was the substitute jump master opened the jump hole—a square hole in the bottom of the Lancaster bomber—and told us to take up jump positions. I was number one, by choice; I have always hated to wait in line. I sat with my feet through the hole, feeling the pressure of the rushing air. Thouville sat with his legs around my bottom, then Franklin, then the O-group. I glanced down through the hole, and there below, beautiful by the light of the full moon, was occupied France.

We droned on, circling. Obviously, the pilot and the navigator were having trouble finding the Dee Zed. "*J'ai une trouille noire,*" Thouville muttered into my ear. I was glad he was in a little black hole. So was I. So was the R.A.F. corporal who was supposed to act as jump master.

The jump master controls the jump, which in a combat situation should be very fast, so that the jumpers are close together for mutual defense. The routine is—or was—for the jump master to shout "Action stations!" as the plane approaches the Dee Zed; then "Running in!" to warn that the jump is imminent; then "Number one, *go;* number two, *go;* number three, *go*" and so on, often with a kick or a push to encourage the hesitant.

"Look, chaps," said the R.A.F. corporal nervously, over the roar of the motors. "I've never done this before, and I

291

don't want to get it wrong. The pilot will light a red light when we're over the Dee Zed. So just as soon as you see a light, Number One, off you go, and the rest of you chaps follow as quick as you can. All right?"

The plane circled more steeply; obviously the pilot and the navigator thought they were near the Dee Zed, but they couldn't find the maquis reception committee's lights. It was getting late—after two in the morning—and if we didn't find the Dee Zed soon we would have to turn back for England. It would be suicide for a slow Lancaster to fly back over the Normandy beachhead in daylight.

My feet dangled in the chilly air. My hands were on the back of the hole, tensed to push when I saw the light. We flew on and on and on. Then, right in front of me, a light flashed on, and I pushed hard with both hands.

I felt the sudden rush of the prop wash. I turned over in the air and my parachute opened and I began to sway down through the moonlit night. I looked up and saw the plane disappearing in the night sky and knew instantly that something was wrong. I could see no friendly parachutes following me down. Below, there were no fires to mark the Dee Zed. The descent was taking too long—we were supposed to jump at eight hundred feet, seconds from the ground. The prop wash had hit me too hard—the plane should have been at stalling speed. And the light had not been red—it had been white. (Later I learned that the nervous R.A.F. corporal, desperate for a cigarette, had lit a flashlight to look for one, and when I jumped he stopped the others.) Even before I reached the ground, I realized two things—that I had been a damn fool, and that I was all alone in occupied France.

My landing was a marvel. A parachute landing is sometimes hard enough to break an ankle, but I landed so lightly that my toes barely touched the ground. I looked up and saw why. My parachute was neatly draped over a small tree, which happened to be just the right height for my soft landing.

I punched the release, and freed myself from the chute, and grabbed the risers, to pull the chute free of the tree and bury it. (We had been sternly warned at Milton Hall to bury our chutes; otherwise the Germans would spot our positions.) I pulled hard. The chute held firm. I went to the other side of the tree and pulled hard again. The tree gave a little, but the chute held fast. There was no way to free the chute from the tree, and by dawn it would be a beacon advertising where I had landed.

I went to the top of a little knoll and sat down behind a bush and tried to think sensibly. I took a healthy swig of brandy from the pocket-sized flask thoughtfully provided by the British army for such occasions. (I still have the flask —I regard it as a talisman and never travel without it.) I cupped a cigarette in my hands (for might there not be Germans about?) and puffed hungrily (I had one pack— only nineteen to go) and thought about what to do next.

In a valley a few hundred yards away, I could make out a village in the moonlight. I would go to the village, I decided, and knock on a door, and ask for help; lots of airmen had been helped by French villagers. I ground out the cigarette, took another pull at the flask, and started off toward the village. As I approached it, a dog barked, then another. I took a few more hesitant steps toward the village, and what sounded like a hundred-dog chorus broke out.

Kee-rist, I thought, how can the Germans help hearing that noise? I retreated to my now-familiar bush, and the canine cacophony slowly faded. I finished the brandy in my flask and cupped another cigarette in my hands (eigh-

293

teen to go) and considered my situation. I was entirely alone in occupied France. I was in American army uniform. I had no idea where I was.

"Face it, Alsop," I said. "You're in trouble."

I started walking in the direction the plane was taking when it disappeared—I could think of nothing better to do —when I saw three trucks winding along a road near the dog-filled village. Gestapo, I thought to myself. Then I heard someone calling my name: "Stewart, Stewart!" I thought, My God, the Gestapo is efficient. They know my first name already. Then I recognized Richard Thouville's voice.

Thouville, Franklin, and the O-group had parachuted to a Dee Zed about ten miles south of where I had so foolishly jumped. The maquis reception committee boasted three trucks, mysteriously propelled by charcoal, and Thouville had organized a search party. By dawn's early light, we were all happily ensconced in the basement of a small chateau, drinking lots of red wine and being embraced by pretty girls.

We spent a couple of months with the maquis thereafter. We assisted in the liberation of several towns, ending conveniently in Cognac, where we consumed vast quantities of *le vrai Napoleon*. There were a few moments of fear, exhaustion, and even some danger, but for the most part those weeks in the maquis were a lot of fun—in some ways the best fun I've had in my life.

When I first made contact with the U.S. Army, I got into a spot of trouble. By September our maquis was thoroughly motorized with Renaults, Peugeots, and even one primitive tank captured from the Italians. But gasoline was a real problem—the gazogenes, powered by charcoal, were wholly unreliable. As there were still a few battalions of Germans holed up in our area, to justify our continued existence, I was sent north to beg some gas from the Americans.

My strange request was referred to a rear-echelon light colonel. I saluted smartly, palm out, clicked my heels, and announced, "Leftenant Alsop reporting, *sir!*"

This was the way I had been taught in the British army to greet a superior officer. The light colonel gave me a lynx-eyed look, taking in brother John's ill-fitting and by this time bedraggled uniform. There had been reports of Germans being sent to France in imitation American uniforms to assassinate General Eisenhower and other key men.

"*Loo*tenant," he said, emphasizing the first syllable, "how come you got your bars the wrong way round?"

"Do I, sir? Sorry, sir," I said. What else was there to say?

"And how come you got your crossed rifles upside down?"

"Sorry, sir," I said, nonplussed. The light colonel lifted a field telephone and asked for counterintelligence.

I had visions of being stood up against a wall, offered a last cigarette, and shot as a German spy. But some phone calls later, my bona fides as "one of those goddam OSS screwballs" was established, and I even got some gas to take back with me to the maquis. So that trouble, like other troubles I have had from time to time, faded away.

But I *was* in trouble, real trouble, that night when I found myself alone in occupied France. A few weeks after I'd got back home, I got in the mail a handsome scroll awarding me a Croix de Guerre with Palme, marked—in type —"Signé, Charles de Gaulle." The citation, I must modestly note, was written by Thouville (I tried to get him an American decoration, but as a new boy with OSS I failed). It reads, in part: *"S'est trouvé de nombreuses fois dans les situations les plus périleuses d'où il s'est toujours sorti avec un calme édifiant et une volonté galvanisante les énergies de tous ceux qui l'entourait."*

295

I cannot boast that my calm is edifying or my will galvanizing, but my situation is undoubtedly again a bit perilous. I came out of that peculiar experience all in one piece, and maybe I will again. Even if my stay of execution turns out to be a short one, I have reason to be grateful, for a happy marriage and a reasonably long, amusing, and interesting life. I even have some reason to be grateful for the experience I have had since that June day when I climbed to the top of the dump at Needwood and realized that I was again in trouble. There have been times when I have been, like Thouville that night over occupied France, in a little black hole. But there have been useful lessons to be learned from the experience.

It is useful, for example, to learn that most people are nicer than they seem to be. It is also useful to know that, although it can be very hard at first, in time one becomes accustomed to living with Uncle Thanatos. One comes to terms with death.

This is being written in late May 1973, in one of NIH's drearily familiar hospital rooms (except for the reproductions from the National Gallery of Art opposite each bed, they are all exactly alike). I came here, on John Glick's orders, a week ago, on May 19.

On Friday, May 18, Joe and Candy flew down from Boston—which they may be leaving soon, since Intercomp has been sold to a California computer company—for a Needwood weekend. Ian and Jill, who are back from Katmandu with a treasure trove of Himalayan artifacts to sell, were to join us on Sunday. On Saturday Joe drove us to Needwood in Tish's station wagon, with me in the front seat and Tish and Candy and Nicky and Andrew squeezed into the back. Andrew was supposed to sit in front, but he is still deeply in love with Candy and insisted on sitting on her lap all the way.

I felt queer on the way out. In fact, I had been feeling queer for some two months. Since mid-March, I had been having those familiar atypical symptoms, night sweats and low-grade fevers, the same unexplained symptoms I had had in September 1971 and intermittently since. But I felt especially queer on Saturday, so when we got to Needwood I went to bed. About five in the afternoon I woke up, feeling not queer but sick, really sick. I took my temperature, and it was over 104. We called John Glick, and he ordered me into NIH. By eight that night, after thumping my back and peering at a chest X ray, he had made his diagnosis— pneumonia again.

In the two months of night sweats and fevers, my blood counts had sunk inexorably. I needed hemoglobin transfusions more frequently than before, and my poor brother Joe had had to join forces with Bob Park as a platelet donor, spending three to six hours of every busy week with a needle in his arm in the plasma pharesis laboratory. But the worst of my counts was the granulocyte count. For weeks it had been 100 or less. Statistically and medically, I was an easy mark for a galloping infection, the kind that kills a leukemic in a matter of hours.

I felt very sick on Saturday night, and I had a feeling, quite a strong feeling, that this time I would not leave NIH on my two feet; that this was what the Bible calls "the end of the days." Given my counts, this was not at all an irrational feeling. But I seem to have been wrong. As this is written, a week after being admitted, I have had no temperature for forty-eight hours, for the first time in more than eight weeks, and John Glick reports that the pneumonia is contained. He is very complimentary about my granulocytes, which,

297

though few in number, seem to be brave and resourceful; John compares them to Napoleon's Old Guard. The granulocytic Old Guard could not have saved me, of course, without the cidal antibiotics that are dripping into my left arm as I type. In any case, I seem to have had yet another stay of execution.

John Glick can make no prognosis about what may happen next. Perhaps I shall drift back into the fever-and-night-sweats routine. Perhaps, as after the October pneumonia, I shall make a halfway comeback, with no fever and feeling reasonably well as long as I get my hemoglobin and platelet transfusions. And just perhaps, although miracles, like lightning, rarely strike twice in the same place, I shall have another remission, as I had after my bout of flu in the autumn of 1971.

In any case, one contrast strikes me. At the beginning of this book, I described the trapped and desperate feeling that came over me after I had been told that I would die quite soon. Last Saturday night, when I felt so sick, I felt rather sure that I would die quite soon, and perhaps very soon, within the next day or so. I did not at all welcome the prospect, but it filled me with no sense of panic. I kissed Tish a fond good night at ten, took some Benadryl, and went easily off to sleep. Why the difference?

Perhaps the state of the nation has something—a very little something—to do with the difference. For weeks now I have been haunted and depressed by a sense that the American system, in which I have always believed in an unquestioning sort of way, the way a boy believes in his family, really is falling apart; by a sense that we are a failed nation, a failed people. And Watergate is surely a peculiarly depressing way to say farewell to all our greatness. It is a whimper—a sleazy little whimper, a grubby little whimper—rather than a bang.

The thought has occurred to me quite often in recent weeks that perhaps this is a good time to bow out. No doubt it was the state of Alsop, far more than the state of the nation, that caused this thought to occur to me so often. The fact is that I have been depressed, the more so because John Glick, on whom I have become excessively dependent, leaves in a few weeks to take up a new post in California. Moreover, I have been feeling lousy.

Since mid-March, when the fevers and the night sweats began, I have written my column for *Newsweek* and worked on this book and driven downtown to dictate letters to Amanda, make telephone calls, and make dates for business lunches. Tish and I, as usual better guests than hosts, have gone out to dinner several times a week and talked and laughed with friends. I have lived, in short, what John Glick calls "a normal life."

But it has not been altogether normal. It is not normal to wake up every night just before dawn, with a fever of 101 or so, take a couple of pills, and settle down to sweat like a hog for four or five hours. It is not normal to feel so weak you can't play tennis or go trout fishing. And it is not normal either to feel a sort of creeping weariness and a sense of being terribly dependent, like a vampire, on the blood of others. After eight weeks of this kind of "normal" life, the thought of death loses some of its terrors.

But the most important reason why I felt no panic fear last Saturday was, I think, the strange, unconscious, indescribable process which I have tried to describe in this book —the process of adjustment whereby one comes to terms with death. A dying man needs to die, as a sleepy man needs to sleep, and there comes a time when it is wrong, as well as useless, to resist.

There was a time, after I first got sick, when I liked to recall another of my small collection of Churchillisms, the familiar story of how Churchill visited his old school, Harrow, in his extreme old age, and the headmaster asked him to say a few words to the boys.

"Never give up," Churchill said. "Never. Never. Never. Never." There is no doubt that the old man lived beyond his allotted span by a tremendous effort of a tremendous will. He lived so long because he never gave up. But to what good end?

I saw Churchill once again, after that luncheon at Chartwell. A year or so before he died, I was in the visitors' gallery of the House of Commons on a reporting trip to London when Sir Winston unexpectedly appeared on the floor. There was a hush as the old man waddled feebly toward his accustomed seat, hunched over and uncertain of every step. He sat down heavily and looked around the House, owlishly, unseeing, as if for some long-vanished familiar face, and then, as the debate resumed, his big head slumped forward grotesquely on his chest. He was an empty husk of a man, all the wit and elegance and greatness drained out of him by age. Like my mother, he should have died herebefore.

There is a time to live, but there is also a time to die. That time has not yet come for me. But it will. It will come for all of us.

Appendix

Memorandum to Stewart Alsop

September 8, 1972

Mr. Stewart Alsop, a white male journalist, then 57 years old, presented to the National Cancer Institute, National Institutes of Health, on July 21, 1971, with a 2-month history of fatigue, dyspnea on exertion, and easy bruiseability. On admission to the National Institutes of Health, he was found to have a normal physical examination. Extensive laboratory evaluations were undertaken after the patient was found to be pancytopenic on admission. His initial blood counts included a hemoglobin of 6.8 gm. %, hematocrit of 19.6%, a retic count of 1.7%, WBC of 1100 with 14% neutrophils, 82% lymphocytes, 3% monocytes, and 1% eosinophils. No blasts were seen on peripheral smear. RBC morphology was normal. His initial platelet count was 20,000. All blood chemistries including renal and liver function tests were within normal limits. His uric acid and LDH were within normal limits. Protein electrophoresis and immunoglobulins were within normal limits. Bone marrow aspiration and biopsy revealed a hypocellular marrow with markedly decreased megakaryocytes, mildly megaloblastic erythroid elements, and 40% abnormal cells. These abnormal cells appeared to be blasts of the leukemic type, but further classification into either myeloblasts or lymphoblasts was impossible. Detailed histochemical, genetic and electron microscopic studies did not provide a definitive answer to the exact nature of these clearly abnormal cells. Cytogenetic studies of both his bone marrow and peripheral blood were normal. Complete metastatic workup was negative. A workup for tuberculosis, collagen disease and dysproteinemia was also negative. Studies for PNH and other forms of hemolysis were negative. B-12, folate and iron studies were within normal limits. Our diagnosis at the time of admission was pancytopenia—probable smoldering leukemia (smoldering leukemia being synonymous with subacute leukemia or aleukemic leukemia).

During the first month after admission there was no progression of his disease—the abnormal cells in his marrow remained approximately 40%, and his peripheral counts remained in the pancytopenic stage as previously mentioned. He was discharged home and resumed work.

Approximately two months after his initial diagnosis he had a brief febrile illness with flu-like symptoms. Complete viral, bacterial, fungal, parasitic and tuberculin cultures were negative. Because of the fever in conjunction with granulocytopenia, he received an 8-day course of antibiotics during which time he became afebrile. During this illness his allopurinol was stopped. It should be noted that he had been on allopurinol for approximately two years prior to his initial NIH admission. This medication had been prescribed by his private physician for mild hyperuricemia. In fact, at NIH, comprehensive evaluation as to his uric acid status revealed that he had mild Type IV Hyperlipidemia. This would account for the previously documented mild elevation in uric acid. With appropriate diet his cholesterol, triglycerides and uric acid returned to normal.

Within one month of this previously mentioned febrile illness his peripheral counts were returning towards normal and bone marrow examination revealed only 6% of these abnormal cells. He received no chemotherapy, and this remis-

304

sion was felt most likely to be spontaneous. The question initially arose whether discontinuing the allopurinol had anything to do with causing the remission. For the next approximately 2 months he continued with normal peripheral counts and bone marrows showing only 7% of these abnormal cells. However, by February 1972, his platelet count and granulocyte count were again failing, and he had 17% of these abnormal cells in his marrow. Therefore, the allopurinol was felt to have played no part in the previously described remission. He continued to feel well throughout this period with a normal physical examination. By May 1972, he had 40% abnormal cells in his marrow, and was requiring platelet and red blood cell transfusions. We have been able to adequately maintain his platelet count by the use of HL-A matched platelets from random donors.

In June and again in July a course of Poly I:C was given, probably without effect.

As of this date he continues to feel well, is working, has a normal physical examination. He remains pancytopenic, receiving platelets once a week and red blood cells once a month. His most recent marrow shows 30% of these abnormal cells. Our diagnosis is that Mr. Alsop has smoldering leukemia, which has remained stable for the past four months. We anticipate giving him a trial of prednisone in the near future.

John H. Glick, M.D.
Clinical Associate
Hematology and Supportive Care Service
National Cancer Institute
National Institutes of Health
Bethesda, Maryland

305

The following is the memorandum Henry Kissinger brought back from Moscow:

U S S R
Academy of Medical Sciences
Institute of Experimental and Clinical Oncology

Moscow 115478, Kashirskoje shosse, 6   Telefone 111 83 42

September 11, 1972

It may be concluded from the medical record received that the patient suffers from the aleukemic variant of acute leukemia. In view of the fact that pancytopenia is revealed by peripheral blood analyses, the only treatment that may be recommended to the patient is that with corticosteroid hormones (prednisolon 1 mg/kg) in combination with symptomatic remedies (antibiotics, haemotransfusions).

The consultant of this case was Prof. Y. I. Lorie.

Acting Deputy Director
for Medical Treatment

(L. Chebotarewa)

Index

307

Alsop, Stewart (*continued*)
16, 56–60, 287–290; family of, 20–21, 185–202, 227; as journalist, 91, 96–97, 103–110, 237–243; political leanings, 90–91, 93, 243; religious leanings, 149–150, 181, 220; World War II service, 16, 32, 35–37, 123–129, 282–295
—illness of: diagnostic problems, 24, 44, 67–68, 77–81, 85–86, 121–122, 143–144, 174–175, 180, 205, 221, 233, 244–245; first symptoms, 15, 17, 25–26, 41, 303; initial AML diagnosis, 9, 22, 24–25, 33, 44, 47, 77, 85, 121–122; low-grade fever and night sweat symptoms, 119, 154, 297–299; near-remission, 139–148, 152–153, 254, 266–267, 304–305; pancytopenia diagnosed, 85, 304, 305; prognosis, 269–270; recrudescence, 209–210, 243–244, 249; smoldering leukemia diagnosis, 10, 180, 205, 209, 254, 304, 305 (*see also* Blood counts; Marrow tests)
—treatment problems, 255, 263–266; chemotherapy rejected, 44, 132, 146, 204, 206, 221, 235, 265–266; immunotherapy ruled out, 209–210, 222; Poly I:C used, 266–269, 305; steroids considered, 244–245, 249, 254–255, 305–306 (*see also* Blood transfusions)
Alsop, Stewart (author's son), 21, 196, 198–200, 201, 275
Alsop, Susan Mary, 20, 21
AML. *See* Acute myeloblastic leukemia
Anemia, 15, 17; aplastic, 18, 67, 153
Anjain, Lekoj, 278–281
Antibiotics, 45, 46, 47, 82, 130
Aplastic anemia, 18, 67, 153
Aspirin, 18, 119, 155
Atlantic, The, 91, 248
Atromid, 153, 181
Attwood, Bill, 134
Auer rods, 205
Auerbach, Stuart, 119
Auto-immunity, 204, 206, 222

Baldwin, Rosie, 173, 174
Barnes, Tracy, 223–224
Bartlett, Charles, 215, 255
Baruch, Bernard, 73, 150
Bay of Pigs operation, 223
BCG vaccine, 202, 203, 209–210

Belloc, Hilaire, 65, 169
Benzine, 18, 25
Biddle, Anthony J. D., Jr., 36–37
Biddle, Francis, 170
Bikini Island, H-bomb test, 278–279
Biopsies, 30, 81, 175
Bissell, Richard, 223
Blasts (abnormal cells), 81–82, 204–205; in immunotherapy, 210
Bleeding: danger in Alsop case, 43, 102, 231, 234, 273; danger to leukemics, 42, 102, 218; platelet control of, 26, 42
Blood cells. *See* Granulocytes; Hemoglobin; Platelets; White blood cells
Blood counts, 39–44; allopurinol and, 120, 145; in Alsop case, 24, 40, 42–44, 81–82, 85, 114, 120, 131–132, 139–142, 144, 207, 212, 232, 235–236, 249, 297, 303–305; minimum safe granulocyte level, 44; minimum safe hemoglobin level, 41; minimum safe platelet level, 42; normal hemoglobin level, 41; normal platelet level, 42; normal white cell level, 43–44; typical AML case, 24, 26, 85; typical AML platelet count, 26; typical AML white count, 24, 26
Blood transfusions, 42–43, 179; allergic reactions to, 122; during chemotherapy, 27; hemoglobin, 27, 41–42, 46; and hepatitis, 42, 43, 271; platelet, 27, 42, 43, 46, 179, 180, 271–277; platelet matching, 179, 274; red blood matching, 42; rejection, 46, 179, 274–275; white cell (leukocyte), 45–46, 179–180
Bohlen, Charles E., 215
Braden, Joan, 233, 237, 247–248
Braden, Thomas, 102, 126–128, 233, 237
Bradlee, Ben, 157–158
Bundy, McGeorge, 170, 171
Bundy, William, 170, 171
Burns, Robert, 217

Cancer: false, drug-induced, 154; leukemia compared to other types, 218; marrow, kinds of, 24, 77–78; question of candor with patients, 51, 82–84, 222, 232, 234; prospects for general cure, 145, 180
Carbone, Dr. (NIH), 254

309

310

Miller, Dr. (NIH), 256
Muskie, Edmund, 104, 115, 158
Myeloblasts, 85, 143, 203–204; Auer rods, 205; doubling time, 175; in normal marrow, 143

National Institutes of Health (NIH), 10, 22–23, 44, 46, 77–78, 111–112, 263; laminar flow rooms, 27–28, 52, 131; leukemia ward, 52, 61; platelet matching work at, 274–277; policy of aggressive treatment, 83; policy of candor with patients, 51, 83–85, 222; as research institute, 84; rules for admission, 51, 83
Needwood Forest (Alsop home), 15, 88, 94, 97–100
New Left, the, 240, 241–242
New York Herald Tribune Syndicate, 70, 96
New York Times, 90, 181; *Magazine*, 61
Newsweek, 10, 17, 41, 55, 80, 90, 100, 156, 159, 173, 178, 242, 268, 299
NIH. *See* National Institutes of Health
Nitze, Paul, 227–228, 229
Nixon, Richard M., 61–62, 98, 105, 106, 107, 128, 234, 242, 248, 269
Nuclear weapons, 281; fallout, 278–279; great power balance, 69, 273

O'Doherty, Kieran, 243
Olson, Culbert, 70–71
Osler, Sir William, 82, 271

Pancytopenia, 80, 85, 153, 304
Paris summit conference, 1960, 216
Payson, Joan, 156
"Peace of mutual terror," Churchill quote, 69, 75–76
Perry, Dr. Richard, 16–24
Petechiae, 273
Platelet matching, 179, 274–277
Platelets, 26, 27; aspirin and, 119, 155; function of, 26, 42; minimum safe level, 42; normal count, 42; production of, 47, 132; transfusions, 27, 42, 43, 46, 179, 180, 271–277; in typical AML case, 26
Polecat Park (Alsop home), 95, 97, 98, 100, 195
Political journalism, 96, 103–110, 157, 181–182, 237–243; thumbsucker columns, 103–104
Political polling, 106–110

Polling, Jim, 159
Poly I:C treatment, 266–269, 305
POMP (drug combination), 245
Presidential elections: of 1952, 106; of 1956, 106–107; of 1960, 108–110; of 1968, 242; of 1972, 234

Ranfurley, Lady Hermione, 284
Raskin, Hy, 104
Realist, The, 241
Red blood cells. *See* Hemoglobin
Remission, in leukemia: chemotherapy-induced, 27, 28–29, 52–53, 86, 123; partial, in Alsop case, 139–148, 152–153, 254, 266–267, 304–305; spontaneous, 86, 153; viremia-induced, 153, 266–267
Ridder, Walter, 106
Roche, John, 158
Roosevelt, Eleanor, 35, 36–38
Roosevelt, Franklin D., 35, 37–38, 68, 73, 89, 91, 98, 169–170, 171, 290
Roosevelt, Quentin, 250
Roosevelt, Theodore, 34, 55, 91–92, 151, 218, 250
Roosevelt, Theodore, Jr., 71, 282
Rosenthal, Dr. Allen, 120, 152–155
Rubin, Jerry, 241, 242
Ruckelshaus, William, 229
Rusk, Dean, 216

Sanderson, Sandy, 83
Saturday Evening Post, 44, 54, 55, 88, 97, 142, 215, 238
Schlesinger, Arthur, Jr., 104
Shultz, George, 171
Sloan Kettering Institute, 174
Smoldering leukemia, 10, 180, 205, 209, 254, 304, 305; survival prognosis, 10, 209
Sommers, Martin, 142
Soviet Union, 75, 216, 262, 269–270; and nuclear balance, 69, 223; Oncology Institute, 270, 306
Special Air Services, 123, 284–286
Spicules, defined, 30
Spleen enlargement: in AML, 85; in dysproteinemia, 175
Sterne, Laurence, 52
Steroid drugs, 244–245, 249, 254–255
Stevenson, Adlai, 106–107
Subacute leukemia, 254, 304. *See also* Smoldering leukemia
Suez crisis of 1956, 170–171
Sulzberger, Cy, 134